THE FORGETTING

ALSO BY DAVID SHENK

The End of Patience

Data Smog

THE FORGETTING

ALZHEIMER'S: PORTRAIT OF AN EPIDEMIC

∾

David Shenk

DOUBLEDAY

New York   London   Toronto   Sydney   Auckland

PUBLISHED BY DOUBLEDAY
a division of Random House, Inc.
1540 Broadway, New York, New York 10036

DOUBLEDAY and the portrayal of an anchor with a dolphin are
trademarks of Doubleday, a division of Random House, Inc.

Several of the names and identifying characteristics of the
individuals depicted in this book have been changed to protect
their privacy.

Library of Congress Cataloging-in-Publication Data
Shenk, David.
The forgetting: Alzheimer's: portrait of an
epidemic / David Shenk.—1st ed.
        p.   cm.
Includes index.
1. Alzheimer's disease.   I. Title.
RC523.2 .S535 2001
616.8'31—dc21   2001028012

ISBN 0-385-49837-3

CONTENTS

᧐

Prologue   *1*

Contents

PART III

END STAGE

THE FORGETTING

❧

LEAR: Does any here know me? This is not Lear.

Does Lear walk thus, speak thus? Where are his eyes?

Either his notion weakens, his discernings

Are lethargied—Ha! Waking? 'Tis not so.

Who is it that can tell me who I am?

FOOL: Lear's shadow.

—William Shakespeare, *King Lear*

PROLOGUE

 ❧

"When I was younger," Mark Twain quipped near the end of his life, "I could remember anything, whether it had happened or not; but my faculties are decaying now and soon I shall be so I cannot remember any but the things that never happened."

At age seventy-two, Twain's memory and wit were intact. But behind his remark lay a grim recollection of another celebrated writer's true decline. In December 1877, Twain had come to Boston at the invitation of William Dean Howells, editor of the *Atlantic Monthly*, to satirize a group of Brahmin intellectuals. Among Twain's targets that night was the father of American Transcendentalism, Ralph Waldo Emerson.

It was after midnight when Twain finally took to the floor at the Hotel Brunswick to spin his yarn. He told the venerable crowd about a lonely miner who had been victimized by three tramps claiming to be famous American writers. The literary outlaws stormed into the miner's cabin, ate his beans and bacon, guzzled his whiskey, and stole his only pair of boots. They played cards and fought bitterly. One of the tramps called himself Emerson.

The point of the skit was to poke some harmless fun at Emerson by corrupting some of his noble expressions. As they played cards at the climax of the story, the Emerson hobo spat out contorted fragments of his poem "Brahma." A mystical paean to immortality, the original included these stanzas:

If the red slayer think he slays,
Or if the slain think he is slain,
They know not well the subtle ways
I keep, and pass, and turn again.

They reckon ill who leave me out;
When me they fly, I am the wings;
I am the doubter and the doubt,
And I the hymn the Brahmin sings.

Twain twisted the verse into drunken poker banter:

I am the doubter and the doubt—
They reckon ill who leave me out,
They know not well the subtle ways I keep,
I pass and deal again.

An elegant master of spoof, Twain was revered around the world as the funniest living man. But on this important night, his material bombed. From the start, Twain drew only silence and quizzical looks, most prominently from Emerson himself. At the finish, Twain later recalled, there "fell a silence weighing many tons to the square inch." He was humiliated. Shortly afterward, he sent a letter of apology to Emerson.

Only then did Twain learn of the hidden backdrop to his performance: Emerson had been present only in body, not in mind. Emerson's dead silence and flat affect, Twain discovered, was a function of neither offense nor boredom. As his daughter Ellen wrote to Twain in reply, it was simply that he had not understood a word of what Twain was saying.

At age seventy-four, this was no longer the Ralph Waldo Emerson who had written "Self-Reliance" and *Nature;* who had said, "Insist on yourself; never imitate"; who had mentored Henry David Thoreau; the Emerson of whom James Russell Lowell had said, "When one meets him the Fall of Adam seems a false report."

This was now a very different man, a waning crescent, caught in the middle stages of a slow, progressive memory disorder that had ravaged his concentration and short-term memory and so dulled his perceptions that he was no longer able to understand what he read or follow a conversation.

"To my father," Ellen wrote to Twain of the performance, "it is as if it had not been; he never quite heard, never quite understood it, and he forgets easily and entirely."

One of the great minds in Western civilization was wasting away inside a still vigorous body, and there was nothing that anyone could hope to do about it.

❧

Taos, New Mexico: March 1999

They came from Melbourne, Mannheim, St. Louis, London, and Kalamazoo; from Lexington, Stockholm, Dallas, Glasgow, Toronto, and Kuopio. From Tokyo, Zurich, and Palo Alto.

Some took two flights, others three or four, followed by a winding three-hour van ride from the floodplains of Albuquerque, up through the high desert terrain of Los Alamos, past the Sandia mountains, past the Jemez volcanic range, past the Camel Rock, Cities of Gold, and OK casinos, up near the foothills of the Sangre de Cristo mountains.

More than two hundred molecular biologists gathered in the small but sprawling city of Taos, amidst the adobe homes and green-chile quesadillas, to share data and hypotheses. This high-altitude, remote desert seemed like a strange place to fight a threatening disease. But specialists at the biannual conference "Molecular Mechanisms in Alzheimer's Disease" needed a refuge from their routine obligations.

For four and a half days they met in Bataan Hall, an old ball-room converted into a civic center. The room had once been used as a shipping-off point for soldiers in World War II, and later named in memory of those same soldiers' wretched ordeal in the infamous Bataan Death March. Some five hundred prisoners died each day on that trek, about the same number now dying each day in the U.S. from Alzheimer's disease.

At 8:00 P.M. on the first evening, Stanley Prusiner, a biologist at the University of California at San Francisco and a 1997 recipient of the Nobel Prize in medicine, rose to give the keynote address. "I can't compete with Monica," he began with a shrug. "But I think we all know that we wouldn't learn anything new."

Barbara Walters' much-anticipated TV interview with Monica Lewinsky was starting to air on ABC at that very moment, which further fueled the sense of isolation. The local support staff had just raced home to their televisions to catch the well-lighted promotion for the million-dollar book about the sordid affair with the needy President.

No TVs here. The scientists in this large, windowless chamber were distracted by something else: Alzheimer's disease was about to become an epidemic. Known as senility for thousands of years, Alzheimer's had only in the past few decades become a major health problem. Five million Americans and perhaps 15 million people worldwide now had the incurable disease, and those numbers would soon look attractive. Beginning in 2011, the first of the baby boomers would turn sixty-five and start to unravel in significant numbers. By 2050, about 15 million people in the U.S. alone would have Alzheimer's, at an annual cost of as much as $700 billion.

Other industrialized nations faced the same trends. In Japan, one in three would be elderly by 2050. In Canada, the number of elderly would increase by 50 percent while the working-age population increased by just 2 percent. "We have to solve this problem, or it's going to overwhelm us," said Zaven Khachaturian, former director of the Alzheimer's Research Office at the National Institutes of Health. Alzheimer's had already become a costly and miserable fixture in society. Unless something was done to stop the disease, it would soon become one of the defining characteristics of civilization, one of the cornerstones of the human experience.

They were here to solve this problem.

PART I

EARLY
STAGE

The other day I was all confused in the street for a split second. I had to ask somebody where I was, and I realized the magnitude of this disease. I realized that this is a whole structure in which a window falls out, and then suddenly before you know it, the whole façade breaks apart.

This is the worst thing that can happen to a thinking person. You can feel yourself, your whole inside and outside, break down.

—M.
New York, New York

Chapter 1

I HAVE LOST MYSELF

❧

A healthy, mature human brain is roughly the size and shape of two adult fists, closed and pressed together at the knuckles. Weighing three pounds, it consists mainly of about a hundred billion nerve cells—neurons—linked to one another in about one hundred *trillion* separate pathways. It is by far the most complicated system known to exist in nature or civilization, a control center for the coordination of breathing, swallowing, pressure, pain, fear, arousal, sensory perception, muscular movement, abstract thought, identity, mood, and a varied suite of memories in a symphony that is partly predetermined and partly adaptable on the fly. The brain is so ridiculously complex, in fact, that in considering it in any depth one can only reasonably wonder why it works so well so much of the time.

Mostly, we don't think about it at all. We simply take this nearly silent, ludicrously powerful electrochemical engine for granted. We feed it, try not to smash it too hard against walls or windshields, and let it work its magic for us.

Only when it begins to fail in some way, only then are we surprised, devastated, and in awe.

On November 25, 1901, a fifty-one-year-old woman with no personal or family history of mental illness was admitted to a psychiatric hospital in Frankfurt, Germany, by her husband, who could no longer ignore or hide quirks and lapses that had overtaken her in recent months. First there were unexplainable bursts of anger, and then a strange series of memory problems. She became increasingly unable to locate things in her own home and began to make surprising mistakes in the kitchen. By the time she arrived at Städtische Irrenanstalt, the Frankfurt Hospital for the Mentally Ill and Epileptics, her condition was as severe as it was curious. The attending doctor, senior physician Alois Alzheimer, began the new file with these notes in the old German Sütterlin script.

She sits on the bed with a helpless expression.
"What is your name?"
Auguste.
"Last name?"
Auguste.
"What is your husband's name?"
Auguste, I think.
"How long have you been here?"
(She seems to be trying to remember.)
Three weeks.

It was her second day in the hospital. Dr. Alzheimer, a thirty-seven-year-old neuropathologist and clinician from the small Bavarian village of Markbreit-am-Main, observed in his new patient a remarkable cluster of symptoms: severe disorientation, reduced comprehension, aphasia (language impairment), paranoia, hallucinations, and a short-term memory so incapacitated that when he spoke her full-name, *Frau Auguste D———*, and asked her to write it down, the patient got only as far as "Frau" before needing the doctor to repeat the rest.

He spoke her name again. She wrote "Augu" and again stopped.

When Alzheimer prompted her a third time, she was able to write her entire first name and the initial "D" before finally giving up, telling the doctor, "I have lost myself."

Her condition did not improve. It became apparent that there was nothing that anyone at this or any other hospital could do for Frau D. except to insure her safety and try to keep her as clean and comfortable as possible for the rest of her days. Over the next four and a half years, she became increasingly disoriented, delusional, and incoherent. She was often hostile.

"Her gestures showed a complete helplessness," Alzheimer later noted in a published report. "She was disoriented as to time and place. From time to time she would state that she did not understand anything, that she felt confused and totally lost. Sometimes she considered the coming of the doctor as an official visit and apologized for not having finished her work, but other times she would start to yell out of the fear that the doctor wanted to operate on her [or] damage her woman's honor. From time to time she was completely delirious, dragging her blankets and sheets to and fro, calling for her husband and daughter, and seeming to have auditory hallucinations. Often she would scream for hours and hours in a horrible voice."

By November 1904, three and a half years into her illness, Auguste D. was bedridden, incontinent, and largely immobile. Occasionally, she busied herself with her bed clothes. Notes from October 1905 indicate that she had become permanently curled up in a fetal position, with her knees drawn up to her chest, muttering but unable to speak, and requiring assistance to be fed.

What was this strange disease that would take an otherwise healthy middle-aged woman and slowly—very slowly, as measured against most disease models—peel away, layer by layer, her ability to remember, to communicate her thoughts and finally to understand the world around her? What most struck Alzheimer, an experienced diagnostician, was that this condition could not fit neatly into any of the standard psychiatric boxes. The symptoms of Auguste D. did not present themselves as a case of acute delirium or the consequence of a stroke; both would have come on more suddenly. Nor was this the general paresis—mood changes, hyperactive reflexes, hallucinations—that can set in during the late stages of syphilis. She was clearly not a victim of dementia praecox (what we now call schizophrenia), or Parkinson's palsy, or Friedreich's ataxia, or Huntington's disease, or Korsakoff's syndrome, or any of the other well-recognized neurological disorders of the day, disorders that Alzheimer routinely treated in his ward. One of the fundamental elements of diagnostic medicine has always been the exercise of exclusion, to systematically rule out whatever can be ruled out and then see what possibilities are left standing. But Alzheimer had nothing left.

What the fifty-one-year-old Auguste D.'s condition did strongly evoke was a well-known ailment among the elderly: a sharp unraveling of memory and mind that had, for more than five thousand years, been accepted by doctors and philosophers as a routine consequence of aging.

History is stacked with colorful, poignant accounts of the elderly behaving in strange ways before they die, losing connection with their memories and the world around them, making rash decisions, acting with the impetuousness and irresponsibility of children. Plato insisted that those suffering from "the influence of extreme old age" should be excused from the commission of the crimes of sacrilege, treachery, and treason. Cicero lamented the folly of "frivolous" old men. Homer, Aristotle, Maimonides, Chaucer, Thackeray, Boswell, Pope, and Swift all wrote of a distressing feebleness of mind that infected those of advancing years.

"Old age," wrote Roger Bacon, "is the home of forgetfulness."

Known as *morosis* in Greek, *oblivio* and *dementia* in Latin, *dotage* in Middle English, *démence* in French, and *fatuity* in eighteenth-century English, the condition was definitively termed *senile dementia* in 1838 by the French psychiatrist Jean Étienne Esquirol. In a depiction any doctor or caregiver would recognize today, Esquirol wrote: "Senile dementia is established slowly. It commences with enfeeblement of memory, particularly the memory of recent impressions."

But that was *senile* dementia. What was this? Alois Alzheimer wanted to know. Why did a fifty-one-year-old appear to be going senile? How could Auguste D. be suffering from the influence of extreme old age?

~

We are the sum of our memories. Everything we know, everything we perceive, every movement we make is shaped by them. "The truth is," Friedrich Nietzsche wrote, "that, in the process by which the human being, in thinking, reflecting, comparing, separating, and combining . . . inside that surrounding misty cloud a bright gleaming beam of light arises, only then, through the power of using the past for living and making history out of what has happened, does a person first become a person."

The Austrian psychiatrist Viktor Frankl made much the same point in *Man's Search for Meaning,* his memoir of experiences as a concentration camp inmate. Frankl recalled trying to lift the spirits of his fellow camp inmates on an especially awful day in Dachau: "I did not only talk of the future and the veil which was drawn over it. I also mentioned the past; all its joys, and how its light shone even in the present darkness. [I quoted] a poet . . . who had written, *Was Du erlebst, kann keine Macht der Welt Dir rauben.* (What you have experienced, no power on earth can take from you.) Not only our experiences, but all we have done, whatever great thoughts we may have had and all we have suffered, all this is not lost, though it is past; we have brought it into being. Having been is a kind of being, and perhaps the surest kind."

Emerson was also fascinated by memory—how it worked, why it failed, the ways it shaped human consciousness. Memory, he offered about a decade or so before his own troubles first appeared, is "the cement, the bitumen, the matrix in which the other faculties are embedded . . . without it all life and thought were an unrelated succession." While he constructed an elaborate external memory system in topical notebooks, filling thousands of pages of facts and observations that were intricately cross-referenced and indexed, Emerson was also known for his own keen internal memory. He could recite by heart all of Milton's "Lycidas" and much of Wordsworth, and made it a regular practice to recite poetry to his children on their walks. His journal entries depict an enchantment with the memory feats of others.

He kept a list:

- Frederic the Great knew every bottle in his cellar.
- Magliabecchi wrote off his book from memory.
- Seneca could say 2,000 words in one hearing.
- L. Scipio knew the name of every man in Rome.
- Judge Parsons knew all his dockets next year.
- Themistocles knew the names of all the Athenians.

"We estimate a man by how much he remembers," Emerson wrote.

Ronald Reagan was never particularly admired for his memory. But in the late 1980s and early '90s, he slowly began to lose his grasp on ordinary function. In 1992, three years after leaving the White House, Reagan's forgetting became impossible to ignore. He was eighty-one.

Both his mother and older brother had experienced senility, and he had demonstrated a mild forgetfulness in the late years of his presidency. Like many people who eventually suffer from the disease, Reagan may have had an inkling for some time of what was to come. In his stable of disarming jokes were several about memory troubles afflicting the elderly. He shared one at a 1985 dinner honoring Senator Russell Long.

An elderly couple was getting ready for bed one night, Reagan told the crowd. The wife turned to her husband and said, "I'm just so hungry for ice cream and there isn't any in the house."

"I'll get you some," her husband offered.

"You're a dear," she said. "Vanilla with chocolate sauce. Write it down—you'll forget."

"I won't forget," he said.

"With whipped cream on top."

"Vanilla with chocolate sauce and whipped cream on top," he repeated.

"And a cherry," she said.

"And a cherry on top."

"Please write it down," she said. "I know you'll forget."

"I won't forget," he insisted. "Vanilla with chocolate sauce, whipped cream, and a cherry on top."

The husband went off and returned after a while with a paper bag, which he handed to his wife in bed. She opened up the bag, and pulled out a ham sandwich.

"I told you to write it down," she said. "You forgot the mustard."

It seems clear enough that Reagan was increasingly bothered by personal memory lapses. In a regular White House checkup late in his second term, the President began by joking to his doctor, "I have three things that I want to tell you today. The first is that I seem to be having a little problem with my memory. I cannot remember the other two."

Did Reagan have Alzheimer's disease in office? Yes and no. Without a doubt, he was on his way to getting the disease, which develops over many years. But it is equally clear that there was not yet nearly enough decline in function to support even a tentative diagnosis. Reagan's mind was well within the realm of normal functioning. Even if his doctors had been looking intently for Alzheimer's, it is still likely that they would not have been able to detect the disease-in-progress. A slight deterioration of memory is so common among the elderly that even today it is considered to be a natural (if unwelcome) consequence of aging. About a third to a half of all human beings experience some mild decline in memory as they get older, taking longer to learn directions, for example, or having some difficulty recalling names or numbers.

Alzheimer's disease overtakes a person very gradually, and for a while can be indistinguishable from such mild memory loss. But eventually the forgetting reaches the stage where it is quite distinct from an absentminded loss of one's glasses or keys. Fleeting moments of almost total confusion seize a person who is otherwise entirely healthy and lucid. Suddenly, on a routine drive home from work, an intersection he has seen a thousand times is now totally unfamiliar. Or he is asking about when his son is coming back from his European vacation, and his wife says: "What do you mean? We both spoke to him last night." Or he is paying the check after a perfectly pleasant night out and it's the strangest thing, but he just cannot calculate the 20 percent tip.

The first few slips get chalked up to anxiety or a lousy night's sleep or a bad cold. But how to consider these incidents of disorientation and confusion when they begin to occur with some frequency? What begin as isolated incidents start to mount and soon become impossible to ignore. In fact, they are not incidents; collectively, they are signs of a degenerative condition. Your brain is under attack. Months and years go by. Now you are losing your balance. Now you can no longer make sense of an analog clock. Now you cannot find the words to complain about your food. Now your handsome young husband has disappeared and a strange elderly man has taken his place. Why is someone taking your clothes off and pouring warm water over you? How long have you been lying in this strange bed?

By 1992, the signs of Reagan's illness were impossible to ignore. At the conclusion of a medical exam in September, as the *New York Times* would later report, Reagan looked up at his doctor of many years with an utterly blank face and said, "What am I supposed to do next?" This time, the doctor knew that something was very wrong.

Sixteen months later, in February 1994, Reagan flew back to Washington, D.C., from his retirement home in Bel Air, California, for what would turn out to be his final visit. The occasion was a dinner celebrating his own eighty-third birthday, attended by Margaret Thatcher and twenty-five hundred other friends and supporters.

Before the gala began, the former President had trouble recognizing a former Secret Service agent whom he had known well in the White House. This didn't come as a total shock to his wife, Nancy, and other close friends, but it did cause them to worry that Reagan might have problems with his speech that night.

The show went on as planned. After an introduction by Thatcher, Reagan strolled to the podium. He began to speak, then stumbled, and paused. His doctor, John Hutton, feared that Reagan was about to humiliate himself. "I was holding my breath, wondering how he would get started," Hutton later recalled, "when suddenly something switched on, his voice resounded, he paused at the right places, and he was his old self."

Back at his hotel after the dinner, Reagan again slipped into his unsettling new self, turning to Nancy and saying, "Well, I've got to wait a minute. I'm not quite sure where I am." Though the diagnosis and public announcement were both months away, Reagan was already well along the sad path already trod by his mother, his brother, and by Auguste D.

The doctors who diagnosed Reagan in 1994 knew with some specificity what was happening to his brain. Portions of his cerebral cortex, the thin layer of gray matter coating the outside of his brain, were becoming steadily clouded with two separate forms of cellular debris: clumpy brown spherical *plaques* floating between the neurons, and long black stringy *tangles* choking neurons from inside their cell membranes. As those plaques and tangles spread, some neurons were losing the ability to transmit messages to one another. Levels of glucose, the brain's sole energy source, were falling precipitously, weakening cell function; neurotransmitters, the chemicals that facilitate messages between the neurons, were becoming obstructed. The tangles in some areas of the brain were getting to be so thick it was like trying to kick a soccer ball through a chain-link fence.

Ultimately, many of the neurons would die, and the brain would begin to shrink. Because the brain is highly specialized, the strangulation of each clump of neurons would restrict a very specific function—the ability to convert recent events into reliable memories, for example, or the ability to recall specific words, or to consider basic math problems. Or, eventually, to speak at all, or recognize a loved one. Or to walk or swallow or breathe.

We know about plaques and tangles because of Auguste D. and Alois Alzheimer. After four and a half years in the hospital, Frau D. died on April 8, 1906. Her file listed the cause as "septicaemia due to decubitis"—acute blood poisoning resulting from infectious bed sores. In her last days, she had pneumonia, inflammation of the kidneys, excessive fluid in the brain, and a high fever. On the day of her death, doctors understood no more than they had on the first day she was admitted. They could say only this about Auguste D.: that a psychic disturbance had developed in the absence of epileptic fits, that the disturbance had progressed, and that death had finally intervened.

Alois Alzheimer wanted to learn more. He wanted to look at her brain.

Standing apart from most doctors at the time, Alzheimer was equally interested in both clinical and laboratory work. He was known for his tireless schedule, his devoted teaching, and his own brand of forgetfulness. An inveterate cigar smoker, he would put a half-smoked cigar down on the table before leaning into a student's microscope for a consultation. A few minutes later, while shuffling to the next microscope, he'd light a fresh cigar, having forgotten about the smoke already in progress. At the end of each day, twenty microscopes later, students recalled, twenty cigar stumps would be left smoldering throughout the room.

But Alzheimer did not forget about the woman who had lost herself in Frankfurt. Though he had since moved to the Royal Psychiatric Clinic, in Munich, to work for the renowned psychiatrist Emil Kraepelin, he sent for Frau D.'s central nervous system as soon as she died. Her brain, brainstem, and spinal cord were gently removed from the elaborate bone casing, that flexible yet durable wrapper that allows us all to crouch, twist, and bump into things without much concern. The exposed contents were then likely wrapped in formalin-soaked towels, packed carefully in a wooden crate, and shipped by locomotive 190 miles southeast to Munich.

Imagine, now, that lifeless brain on a passenger train. A coconut-sized clump of grooved gelatinous flesh; an intricate network of prewired and self-adapting mechanisms perfected over more than a billion years of natural selection; powered by dual chemical and electrical systems, a machine as vulnerable as it is complex, designed to sacrifice durability for maximal function, to burn brightly—a human brain is 2 percent of the body's weight but requires 20 percent of its energy consumption—at the cost of impermanence. Enormously powerful and potato-chip fragile at the same time, the brain is able to collect and retain a universe of knowledge and understanding, even wisdom, but cannot hold on to so much as a phone number once the glucose stops flowing. The train, an elementary device by comparison, can, with proper maintenance, be sustained forever. The brain, which conceived of the train and all of its mechanical cousins, cannot. It is ephemeral by design.

But there was nothing in the brain's blueprint about this sort of thing, as far as Alzheimer could infer. This was a flaw in the design, a molecular glitch, a *disease process,* he suspected, and it was important to see what that process looked like up close.

It was also now actually possible to do this for the first time, thanks to a whirl of European innovation. Ernst Leitz and Carl Zeiss had just invented the first distortion-free microscopes, setting a standard in optics that survives today. Franz Nissl had revolutionized tissue-staining, making various cell constituents stand out, opening up what was characterized as "a new era" in the study of brain cells and tissues. (The "Nissl method" is still in use. Nissl, a close collaborator and friend of Alois Alzheimer, became a medical school legend with his instructions on how to time the staining process. "Take the brain out," he advised. "Put it on the desk. Spit on the floor. When the spit is dry, put the brain in alcohol.")

Dr. Alzheimer's assistants prepared for microscopic examination more than 250 slides from slivers of the outer lining (the meninges) of Frau D.'s brain; from the large cerebral vessels; from the frontal, parietal, and occipital areas of the cerebral cortex (locus of conscious thought); from the cerebellum (regulator of balance, coordination, gait) and the brainstem (breathing and other basic life functions); and from the spinal cord, all chemically preserved in a cocktail of 90 percent alcohol/10 percent formalin, and stained according to a half-dozen recipes of Alzheimer's contemporaries.

Having fixed, frozen, sliced, stained, and pressed the tissue between two thin pieces of glass, Alzheimer put down his cigar and removed his pince-nez spectacles, leaned into his state-of-the-art Zeiss microscope, and peered downward. Then, at a magnification of several hundred times, he finally saw her disease.

It looked like measles, or chicken pox, of the brain. The cortex was speckled with crusty brown clumps—plaques—too many to count. They varied in size, shape, and texture and seemed to be a hodgepodge of granules and short, crooked threads, as if they were sticky magnets for microscopic trash.

The plaques were nestled in amongst the neurons, in a space normally occupied by supporting tissue known as glial cells. They were so prominent that Alzheimer could see them without any stain at all, but they showed up best in a blend of magenta red, indigo carmine, and picric acid. Alzheimer had squinted at thousands of brain slides, but he found these clumps "peculiar" and had no idea what they could be.

A different stain, invented just four years earlier, revealed the other strange invasion of Auguste D.'s brain. In the second and third layers of the cortex, nearly a third of the neurons had been obliterated internally, overrun with what Alzheimer called "a tangled bundle of fibrils"—weedy, menacing strands of rope bundled densely together.

The tangles were just as foreign to Alzheimer as the plaques, but at least the ingredients looked familiar. They seemed to be composed of fibrils, an ordinary component of every neuron. It was as if these mild-mannered, or "Jekyll," fibrils had swallowed some sort of steroidal toxin and been transformed into "Hyde" fibrils, growing well out of proportion and destroying everything within their reach. Many affected neurons were missing a nucleus completely, and most of the rest of their cell contents. A good portion of the neurons in the upper cell layers of the cortex had disappeared. They just weren't there. Alzheimer's assistant Gaetano Perusini wrote of the neurofibrillary tangles in Frau D.'s brain:

> It is impossible to give a description of all the possible pictures: there are present all the variable and twisted formations that one can imagine; at times large fibrils seem to lie only on the periphery of the cell. But on focusing untangled fibrillar agglomerations are found. Changing the focus again one has the impression that the single dark-coloured fibrils unwind into an infinite number of

thinner fibrils ... arranged as balls of twine or half-moons or baskets.

Connecting a camera lucida to the top of the microscope, Alzheimer and Perusini both drew pictures of the tangles.

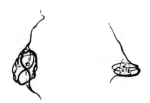

The menacing drawings perfectly convey the ghastly significance of their discovery. Here was the evidence that Auguste D. had not lost herself. Rather, her "self" was taken from her. Cell by cell by cell, she had been strangled by unwelcome, malignant intruders.

What were they, exactly, and where did they come from?

❧

When my kids began to say they were worrying about my memory, I said to them, "Well, I've never had a photographic memory, and I have a lot more on my mind now. There's a lot more to remember with life being so complex. How can I remember everything? What do you want—total recall?" I always had an answer. I really was in denial, and it just didn't occur to me that I had a problem. But I also knew that they weren't totally exaggerating.

—D.
New York, New York

❧

Chapter 2

BOTHERED

❦

Queens, New York: August 1998

It was lunch time in Freund House, in the village of Flushing. A small group of elderly Jews sat quietly at a round table. Not much was said as they ruffled open their brown paper bags and popped the lids off drinks. Someone brought in a big bottle of ginger ale and some plastic cups, and offered to pour.

Irving looked over at Greta and noticed that she was sitting still, her hands folded together on the bright red table cloth.

"Did you bring your lunch today, Greta?"

"I don't think so. I usually don't bring my lunch here."

"Yes, you do. You bring cereal."

Irving waited for Greta to recollect her routine, but she could not. An elegant, shrunken woman with short cropped hair, dark eyebrows, and a supple, leathery face, Greta did not look even remotely like someone in decline. Her eyes still sparkled and her voice had spunk. She spoke without hesitation and in full, clear sentences. There was no clue from her cadences that her brain was under attack.

Paying close attention, though, one could tell that something was not right. For example, in a conversation about Japan, Greta very clearly explained that she had been there a number of times. She discussed the temples of Kyoto, which she enjoyed, and the food, which she did not.

Then, about an hour later, the subject of Japan came up again. This time, she said matter-of-factly, "Japan—never did get there. Couldn't get in."

These hiccups in logic were typical, I now recognized, of someone beginning to advance past the very earliest stages of the disease. She wasn't very far along yet, and most of her brain was still working quite well; but her symptoms were no longer strictly limited to the classic short-term memory loss that usually signals the disease's onset. Occasionally, now, a queer incongruity would creep in.

Standing off to one side of the table was Judy Joseph, the co-leader, with Irving Brickman, of this support group. About a year earlier she had been introduced to Irving in the New York offices of the Alzheimer's Association, where each had come to see what, if anything, could be done about this ominous new social phenomenon. Suddenly, it seemed, Alzheimer's disease was everywhere. Nursing home dementia units were filling beyond capacity. Middle-aged children were moving back home to take care of their parents. Community police were regularly being phoned to help track down wandering relatives. The disease was cropping up continually in newspaper articles and everyday conversation. Perhaps most tellingly, a vibrant Alzheimer's consumer market was springing up—products like automatic medication dispensers (no memory required!), wireless tracking devices for wanderers, and even a stovetop fire extinguisher designed explicitly for people who might forget to turn off the range.

All of a sudden, everyone seemed to know someone touched by Alzheimer's. Partly, this was due to a shift in public conception of senile dementia. Only in the mid-1970s had doctors started to realize that senility is not an inevitable process of brain aging and decay but a recognizable—and perhaps one day treatable—disorder. Gradually, this perception also started to seep into the general consciousness: *Senility is a disease.*

Since then, there had been a staggering rise in actual cases of Alzheimer's, corresponding to a vast increase in the elderly population. People were now living much longer lives. Longer lives meant more cases of Alzheimer's. Since 1975, the estimated number of Alzheimer's cases in the U.S. had grown tenfold, from 500,000 to nearly 5 million. Worldwide, the total was probably about three times that figure. In the absence of a medical breakthrough, the gloomy trend would not only continue, but would also get much, much worse.

The Roman poet Virgil wrote in the first century B.C., "Time wastes all things, the mind, too." He was partly right. Scientists do not believe that Alzheimer's is an *inevitable* consequence of aging. Many people will never get the disease regardless of how long they live. But aging is by far the greatest risk factor. It is almost unheard of in people aged 20–39, and very uncommon (about one in 2,500) for people aged 40–59. For people in their sixties, the odds begin to get more worrisome. An estimated

- 1 percent of 65-year-olds
- 2 percent of 68-year-olds
- 3 percent of 70-year-olds
- 6 percent of 73-year-olds
- 9 percent of 75-year-olds
- 13 percent of 77-year-olds

and so on have Alzheimer's or a closely related dementia. The risk accelerates with age, to the point where dementia affects nearly half of those eighty-five and over.

So, as the twentieth century came to a close, a shadow legacy was rapidly becoming apparent—the dark, unintended consequence of the century's great advances in hygiene, nutrition, and medicine. Life spans in industrialized nations had nearly doubled over the previous one hundred years, and the percentage of elderly among the general population had more than tripled. In the process, the number of cases of senile dementia mushroomed. A hundred years before, it had not even been a statistical blip. Paradoxically, in the full blush of medical progress of the twentieth century, it had blossomed into a major public health problem.

Most strikingly to social workers like Judy and Irving, the number of people who had Alzheimer's *and who knew they had Alzheimer's* had exploded. A huge portion of the newly diagnosed cases were in the very early stages of the disease. "This is something new in the field," Irving explained. "Most people never before realized that there *is* an early stage of Alzheimer's. I had worked with the more advanced stages, but when I came into this it was overwhelming for me. It's very hard to get used to a normal person who happens to have dementia. It's a whole different ballgame."

Judy and Irving recognized, along with many others in the national Alzheimer's community, that something had to be done to help this emerging new constituency: early-stage dementia sufferers still functioning well enough to fully understand what lay ahead. With the assistance of the Alzheimer's Association, they formed a support group at Freund House. "Our goal," explained Irving, "is to try to help these people live a quality life, to help them gain some coping mechanisms for their deficits, and to help them feel better as human beings." While scientists did battle with this disease, victims and their families had the opposite task: to make a certain peace with it, to struggle to understand the loss, come to terms with it, create meaning out of it.

Alzheimer's is what doctors call a disease of "insidious onset," by which they mean that it has no definitive starting point. The plaques and tangles proliferate so slowly—over decades, perhaps—and silently that their damage can be nearly impossible to detect until they have made considerable progress. Part of the function of any early-stage support group must be to try to make sense of this strange new terrain that lies between *healthy* and *demented.* Where, in specific behavioral terms, is the person overshadowed by the disease?

Individually and collectively, the Freund House group was trying to find out, and to make sense of the answer. "My wife gets frustrated with me," Arnie related to his fellow group members, "and she is right to be frustrated. She asks me to put a can in the recycling . . . and I don't do it. She says, 'I know this is because of your illness, that this is not you.' "

Sadie nodded her head in recognition. "My mother had this, too," she said. "Now I know what it was like for my father to take care of her. We used to get so mad at him when he would be short with her."

Coping with a particular disability was one thing; trying to cope with an ever-shifting invisible illness, though, was a challenge unique to Alzheimer's disease. In this early period, the insidiousness itself was often the most troubling thing about the disease—arguably even a disease unto itself. As a group, these new patients could gain a more confident understanding of their disease, and tackle issues that would seem impossibly difficult to one isolated, failing person.

Driving, for instance. The first big question they confronted right after forming the group was: Should they continue, in this blurry period of semi-normalcy, to pilot massive steel boxes at thirty and forty and fifty miles per hour down roads lined with bicycles and toddlers? Studies showed conclusively that Alzheimer's is, overall, a major driving hazard. Bystanders had been killed by Alzheimer's patients making a lapse in judgment or being overcome momentarily by confusion. But the law had not yet caught up with this reality. Even with a diagnosis, no doctor or judge had ever confiscated a license. Families were forced to decide on their own when driving was no longer appropriate.

Together, after much deliberation, the group decided that it had already become too dangerous. Collectively, they gave up this highly charged symbol of autonomy and competence. On this shaky new terrain, a person's independence could no longer be taken for granted.

In the summer of 1984, at the age of eighty-five, E. B. White, the tender essayist and author of *Charlotte's Web,* became waylaid by some form of dementia. It came on very swiftly. In August, he began to complain of some mild disorientation. "We didn't pay much attention," recalls his stepson, Roger Angell, "because he was a world-class hypochondriac." But just a few weeks later, White was severely confused much of the time. By the following May, he was bedridden with full-on dementia, running in and out of vivid hallucinations and telling visitors, "So many dreams—it's hard to pick out the right one." He died just a few months after that, in October 1985.

An obituary in the *New York Times* reported White as having Alzheimer's disease, but that appeared to miss the mark. In fact, he was never even informally diagnosed with the disease, and his symptoms strongly suggested another illness. The rapid onset of the confusion and the abrupt shift from one stage to the next were classic signs of multi-infarct dementia, the second-most common cause (15 percent) of senile dementia after Alzheimer's (60 percent). Multi-infarct dementia is caused by a series of tiny strokes. Its victims can have much in common with those of Alzheimer's, but the experience is not as much of an enigma. Its cause is known, somewhat treatable, and, to a certain extent, preventable (diet, exercise, and medication can have an enormous impact on risk of strokes). Its jerky, stepwise approach is easier to follow and understand as symptoms worsen.

Alzheimer's disease is not abrupt. It sets in so gradually that its beginning is imperceptible. Creeping diseases blur the boundaries in such a way that they can undermine our basic assumptions of illness. Alzheimer's drifts from one stage to the next in a slow-motion haze. The disease is so gradual in its progression that it has come to be formally defined by that insidiousness. This is one of the disease's primary clinical features, one key way that Alzheimer's can be distinguished from other types of dementia: those caused by strokes, brain tumor, underactive thyroid, and vitamin deficiency or imbalance in electrolytes, glucose, or calcium (all treatable and potentially reversible conditions).

It is also nearly impossible to officially diagnose. A definitive determination requires evidence of both plaques and tangles—which cannot be obtained without drilling into the patient's skull, snipping a tiny piece of brain tissue, and examining it under a microscope. Brain biopsies are today considered far too invasive for a patient who does not face imminent danger. Thus—Kafka would have enjoyed this—as a general rule, Alzheimer's sufferers must die before they can be definitively diagnosed. Until autopsy, the formal diagnosis can only be "probable Alzheimer's."

These days, a decent neuropsychologist can maneuver within this paradox—can make a diagnosis of probable Alzheimer's with a confidence of about 90 percent—through a battery of tests. The process almost always begins with this simple quiz:

What is today's date?
What day of the week is it?
What is the season?
What state are we in?
What city?
What neighborhood?
What building are we in?
What floor are we on?
I'm going to name three objects and I want you to repeat
    them back to me: street, banana, hammer.
I'd like you to count backwards from one hundred by
    seven. [Stop after five answers.]

Can you repeat back to me the three objects I mentioned
    a moment ago?

[Points at any object in the room.] What do we call this?

[Points at another object.] What do we call this?

Repeat after me: "No if's, and's, or but's."

Take this piece of paper in your right hand, fold it in half,
    and put it on the floor.

[Without speaking, doctor shows the patient a piece of pa-
    per with "CLOSE YOUR EYES" printed on it.]

Please write a sentence for me. It can say anything at all,
    but make it a complete sentence.

Here is a diagram of two intersecting pentagons. Please
    copy this drawing onto a plain piece of paper.

This neurological obstacle course is called the Mini Mental State Examination (MMSE). Introduced in 1975, it has been a part of the standard diagnostic repertoire ever since. The MMSE is crude but generally very effective in detecting problems with time and place orientation, object registration, abstract thinking, recall, verbal and written cognition, and constructional praxis. A person with normal functioning will score very close to the perfect thirty points (I scored twenty-nine, getting the date wrong). A person with early-to-moderate dementia will generally fall below twenty-four.

The very earliest symptoms in Alzheimer's are short-term memory loss—the profound forgetting of incidents or conversations from just a few hours or the day before; fleeting spatial disorientation; trouble with words and arithmetic; and some impairment of judgment. Later on, in the middle stages of the disease, more severe memory problems are just a part of a full suite of cognitive losses. Following that, the late stages feature further cognitive loss and a series of progressive physical disabilities, ending in death.

One brilliantly simple exam, the Clock Test, can help foretell all of this and can enable a doctor to pinpoint incipient dementia in nine out of ten cases. In the Clock Test, the doctor instructs the patient to draw a clock on a piece of paper and then draw hands to a certain time. Neurologists have discovered that patients in the early stages of dementia tend to make many more errors of omission and misplacing of numbers on the clock than cognitively healthy people. They're not entirely sure why this is, but the accuracy of the test speaks for itself.

A battery of other performance tests can help highlight and clarify neurological deficiencies. The Buschke Selective Reminding Test measures the subject's short-term verbal memory. The Wisconsin Card Sorting Test gauges the ability to deduce sorting patterns. In the Trail Making Test, psychomotor skills are measured by timing a subject's attempt to draw a line connecting consecutively numbered circles. Porteus Mazes measure planning and abstract-puzzle-solving ability.

If the patient performs poorly in a consistent fashion, the next step will likely involve elaborate instruments. Conveniently for physicians, Alzheimer's disease always begins in the same place: a curved, two-inch-long, peapod-like structure in the brain's temporal lobes called the hippocampus (the temporal lobes are located on either side of the head, inward from the ear). Doctors can get a good look at the hippocampus with a magnetic resonance imaging (MRI) scanner, which bombards the body with radio waves and measures the reflections off tissue. A simple volume measurement of the hippocampus will often show, even in the very early stages of Alzheimer's, a pronounced decrease in volume, particularly in contrast with other brain structures. By itself, the MRI cannot diagnose Alzheimer's. But it can add one more helpful piece to the diagnostic puzzle.

Other advanced measurements might also help: A positron emission tomography (PET) scan may detect a decrease in oxygen flow or glucose metabolism in the same area. A single photon emission computed tomography (SPECT) scan may catch decreases in blood flow. A moderate to severe amount of slowing in the alpha rhythm in an electroencephalogram (EEG) is often characteristic of dementia. But such measurements are generally not required for a tentative diagnosis. In the face of convincing results from memory and performance tests, and in the absence of any contravening evidence—disturbance in consciousness, extremely rapid onset of symptoms, preponderance of tremors or other muscular symptoms, difficulties with eye movements or reports of temporary blindness, seizures, depression, psychosis, head trauma, a history of alcoholism or drug abuse, any indication of diabetes, syphilis, or AIDS—a diagnosis of *probable Alzheimer's* is rendered.

Alzheimer's disease. The diagnosis is a side-impact collision of overwhelming force. It seems unreal and unjust. After coming up for air, the sufferer might ask, silently or out loud, "What have I done to deserve this?" The answer is, simply, *nothing.* "I remember walking out of the clinic and into a fresh San Diego night feeling like a very helpless and broken man," recalled Bill, a fifty-four-year-old magazine editor. "I wondered if there was anything for me to live for."

It can take a while to sink in. Experienced doctors know not to try to convey any other important information to a patient or family member on the same day that they disclose the diagnosis. They put some helpful information into a letter, and schedule a follow-up.

There is no cure for Alzheimer's at the present time, and not much in the way of treatment. Historically, the one saving grace of the disease over the years has been that many, if not most, of the people who acquire the disease do not comprehend what is about to happen to them and their families. Now, for better or worse, that has changed. More and more are learning at the earliest possible opportunity what they have, and what it means.

What will they do with the advance knowledge? It is not an easy question. Will they use the time left to get their affairs in order and to prepare themselves emotionally for the long fade? Or will the knowledge only add to the frustration and force them into a psychological spiral to accompany the physiological one?

The Freund House early-stage support group was one experimental approach to tackling such unknowns. When Judy and Irving created it in 1997, they weren't sure it would work. Could people struggling with memory loss, spatial disorientation, and confusion actually strike up a meaningful relationship with a group of strangers? They had to assemble just the right team. "We had to turn many people away," said Judy, "because we didn't feel they were right for a support group. They weren't introspective enough. They weren't *bothered* enough."

The group was also temporary by design. As participants lost the ability to contribute, they would be eased out of the group, and perhaps admitted to a middle-stage group like the one that Judy ran down the hall. In that group, volunteer caregivers always accompanied patients to the restroom and back, because otherwise they would get lost. Most, not all, still responded to their own name. After a cafeteria-style lunch, everyone came together in a circle to sing fun songs together, like the theme from *Barney:*

I love you
You love me
We're a happy family

Members of the early-stage group occasionally caught a glimpse of the middle-stage group as they passed by to get a cup of coffee. The quiet, desperate hope of everyone in this group was not to end up in the other group. Barring a scientific miracle, though, there would be no avoiding it. The average interval from diagnosis to death in Alzheimer's disease is eight years.

In the meantime, there were a hundred small consolations. The early-stage group members had quickly come to rely on one another for help through this very strange ordeal. Sometimes barely able to remember from week to week, they had nevertheless become friends. They shared memories of movie stars and kosher butchers. They talked about travel and passed around pictures of grandchildren. They even talked politics.

"Greta, any comments on Giuliani?" Judy asked one afternoon.

Greta swatted an invisible bug away from her face. "Oh don't get me started about him," she said. "You know I can't stand him."

"Clinton, then? What does everyone think about Monica?"

Opinions ran the gamut. Ted, his hands shaking with a Parkinsonian tremor (it is not unusual for people to suffer from both Parkinson's and Alzheimer's), suggested that Clinton should resign because he lied directly to the American people. Greta, a lifelong subscriber to *The Nation,* thought that Clinton probably kissed Monica but that the whole issue was overblown. Sadie thought it was all a Republican scheme.

Doris had an opinion, too, but with her severe expressive aphasia—an inability to retrieve words—she had great difficulty making it known.

"Gore . . . President . . . I think . . . good leader . . . lies . . ."

She appeared to be aware of her thoughts and very clear on what she wanted to say. But the words were no longer accessible. This was especially painful to watch because, as everyone in the group knew by now, Doris had a forty-year-old son with cerebral palsy who was deaf. The two were very close, and, as it happened, she was the only one in the family to have ever learned sign language. Now Doris's aphasia was also wiping away that second and more vital language. She could no longer speak to her son, leaving him marooned.

It was now a few minutes after one o'clock, time to say goodbye for the week. Rides were arranged. Someone went to fetch William's wife, a volunteer in the middle-stage group.

Robert seemed to be having a hard time of it. Just a moment before, he had been lucidly telling me about his family and his past. He'd had no problem relating how he was spirited out of Nazi Germany as a young boy, turned over to relatives in England and later in New York. I learned all about his children, their occupations and families, the cities they lived in. But now he was struggling to understand a piece of paper his wife had written out for him about getting home. To the undamaged brain, the instructions were fairly straightforward—*Robert will be picked up by the car service at 1:15, and should be driven to his home at* _____

Street. . . . —but he was having a lot of trouble making sense of it. Then there was the other problem. In the last half hour, he had told me how he eventually came to live in the Bronx, where he was introduced to his wife, a distant cousin. He had described how crowded that Bronx apartment was, and where else he had lived in the city as he'd grown older. But now, for the life of him, Robert could not remember where he had put his jacket.

It was on the back of his chair.

Very often I wander around looking for something which I know is very pertinent, but then after a while I forget about what it is I was looking for. . . . Once the idea is lost, everything is lost and I have nothing to do but wander around trying to figure out what it was that was so important earlier. You have to learn to be satisfied with what comes to you.

—C.S.H.
Harrisonburg, Virginia

Chapter 3

THE GOD WHO FORGOT AND
THE MAN WHO COULD NOT

᭶

*There could be no happiness, cheerfulness, hope, pride,
immediacy, without forgetfulness. The person in whom this
apparatus of suppression is damaged, so that it stops working, can
be compared . . . to a dyspeptic; he cannot "cope" with anything.*

—FRIEDRICH NIETZSCHE

As found in the *Pyramid Texts,* from 2800 B.C., *Ra* was the Sun
God, the creator of the universe and of all other gods. From his
own saliva came air and moisture. From his tears came humankind
and the river Nile. He was all-powerful and, of course, immortal—
but still not immune to the ravages of time: Ra, the supreme God,
became old and senile. He began to lose his wits, and became easy
prey for usurpers.

Throughout recorded history, human beings have been celebrating the powers of memory and lamenting its frailties. "Worse

than any loss in body," wrote the Roman poet Juvenal in the first century A.D., "is the failing mind which forgets the names of slaves, and cannot recognize the face of the old friend who dined with him last night, nor those of the children whom he has begotten and brought up."

It took several thousand years, though, for anyone to figure out how memory actually worked. Plato was among the first to suggest a mechanism. His notion was of a literal impression made upon the mind. "Let us suppose," he wrote, "that every man has in his mind a block of wax of various qualities, the gift of Memory, the mother of the Muses; and on this he receives the seal or stamp of those sensations and perceptions which he wishes to remember. That which he succeeds in stamping is remembered and known by him as long as the impression lasts; but that, of which the impression is rubbed out or imperfectly made, is forgotten, and not known."

Later came the ventricular theory of cognition, from Galen (129–ca. 199 A.D.), Nemesius (fourth century), and St. Augustine (354–430). According to this notion, the three major functions of the brain—sensation, movement, and memory—were governed from three large, round fluid-filled sacs. Vital Spirit, a mysterious substance that also contained the human soul, was harbor to the swirl of memories.

From this model came *cerebral localization,* the theory that the various functions of the brain were each controlled by specialized "modules." This model of specialization turned out to be generally correct (if radically different in the details from what Galen had imagined). In the early twentieth century, it emerged that the brain wasn't really an organ so much as a collection of organs, dozens of structures interacting with one another in dazzling complexity. Deep in the center of the brain the amygdala regulates fear while the pituitary coordinates adrenaline and other hormones. Visual stimulus is processed in the occipital lobe, toward the rear of the skull. Perception of texture is mediated by Area One of the parietal lobe near the top of the head, while, just to the rear, the adjacent Area Two differentiates between the size and shape of objects and the position of joints. The prefrontal cortex, snuggled just behind the forehead, spurs self-determination. Broca's area, near the eyes, enables speech. Wernicke's area, above the ears, facilitates the understanding of speech.

The more researchers discovered about localization, though, the more they wondered about the specialized zone for memory. Where was it? If vision was in the back of the brain, texture on top, and so on, what region or regions controlled the formation of lasting impressions and the retrieval of those impressions?

Part of the answer came in 1953, when a Harvard-trained neurosurgeon named William Beecher Scoville performed experimental surgery on a twenty-seven-year-old patient known as H.M. He had been suffering from violent epileptic seizures since childhood, and in a last-ditch effort to give him a chance at a normal life, Scoville removed a small collection of structures, including the hippocampus, from the interior portion of his brain's two temporal lobes. The surgery was a great success in that it significantly reduced the severity of H.M.'s epilepsy. But it was also a catastrophe in that it eliminated his ability to lay down new memories. The case revolutionized the study of memory, revealing that the hippocampus is essential in consolidating immediate thoughts and impressions into longer-lasting memories (which are in turn stored elsewhere).

Time stopped for H.M. in 1953. For the rest of his long life, he was never again able to learn a new name or face, or to remember a single new fact or thought. Many doctors, researchers, and caregivers got to know him quite well in the years that followed, but they were still forced to introduce themselves to him every time they entered his room. As far as H.M. was concerned, he was always a twenty-five-year-old man who was consulting a doctor about his epilepsy (he had also lost all memory of the two years immediately prior to the surgery). H.M. became perhaps the most important neurological subject in history and was subject to a vast number of studies, but he remembered none of the experiments once they were out of his immediate concentration. He was always in the Now.

In the clinical lexicon, this was a perfect case of *anterograde amnesia,* the inability to store any new memories. Persons with incipient Alzheimer's disease exhibit a slightly less severe form of the same problem. The memory of leaving the car keys in the bathroom isn't so much *lost* as it was never actually *formed.*

In a healthy brain, sensory input is converted into memory in three basic stages. Before the input even reaches consciousness, it is held for a fraction of a second in an immediate storage system called a *sensory buffer.*

Moments later, as the perception is given conscious attention, it passes into another very temporary system called *short-term (working) memory.* Information can survive there for seconds or minutes before dissolving away.

Some of the information stirring in working memory is captured by the mechanism that very slowly converts into a *long-term memory* lasting years and even a lifetime.

Long-term memories can be either *episodic* or *semantic.* Episodic memories are very personal memories of firsthand events remembered in order of occurrence. *Before the baseball game the other day, I put on my new pair of sneakers, which I had gotten ear-*

lier that morning. Then we drove to the stadium. Then we parked.
Then we gave the man our tickets. Then we bought some hot dogs.
Then we went to our seats . . .

Now, days later, if I notice a mustard stain on my shoe, I can
plumb my episodic memory to determine when and how it happened. If my feet start bothering me, my episodic memory will
help me figure out whether it happened before or after I bought
my new shoes.

Semantic memories are what we know, as opposed to what we
remember doing. They are our facts about the world, stored in relation to each other and not when we learned them. The memory
of Lincoln being assassinated by John Wilkes Booth is semantic.

They are separate systems—interrelated, but separate. An
early-stage Alzheimer's patient who cannot retain memories of
where she put her keys has not forgotten what keys are for, or what
kind of car she drives. That will come much, much later, when she
starts to lose old semantic memories.

The experience with H.M. taught researchers that the hippocampus is key to long-term memory formation. Without that
tiny organ, he was totally incapable of forming new, lasting memories. Alzheimer's patients suffer the exact same systemic loss, but
over several years rather than one surgical afternoon. For H.M.,
there were no new memories after 1953, period. In later years, he
was unable to recognize his own face in the mirror. Real time had
marched on, 1955 . . . 1962 . . . 1974, but as far as he was concerned, he was still twenty-five years old. If you are a young man,
alert and intelligent, and you look into an ordinary mirror only to
discover the face of a sixty-year-old perfectly mimicking your expressions, perhaps only then do you know the real meaning of the
word *horror.* Fortunately, the extreme distress H.M. suffered dur-

ing such world-shattering incidents was always immediately and completely forgotten as soon as his attention could be distracted by something happening in the new moment. Not remembering can sometimes be a great blessing.

The discovery of hippocampus-as-memory-consolidator was critical. What memory specialists have been trying to figure out ever since then is, once formed, where do these long-term memories actually reside? Are memories stored up in the front of the brain in the prefrontal cortex? On top, in the parietal lobe? In the brainstem at the base of the brain? Where?

One tantalizing theory emerged in the late 1950s: memories were everywhere, stored in discrete molecules scattered throughout the brain. A stampede to confirm this notion was set off by a 1962 *Journal of Neuropsychiatry* article, "Memory Transfer Through Cannibalism in Planaria," in which the University of Michigan's James McConnell eagerly reported that worms could capture specific memories of other worms simply by eating those worms. McConnell had trained a group of flatworms to respond to light in a noninstinctive way. He then killed these worms, chopped them up, and fed them to untrained flatworms. After eating their brethren, McConnell claimed, the untrained worms proceeded to behave as though they had been trained—they had somehow acquired the memory of the trained worms. It was the unexpected apotheosis of the old saying, "You are what you eat."

Out of this report numerous research grants were born, some of which yielded tantalizing results. Three years after McConnell's initial study, four California scientists reported in the journal *Science* that when cells extracted from the brains of trained rats were injected into the guts of untrained rats, the untrained rats picked up the learned behavior of the trained rats. These experiments apparently showed that specific, concrete individual memories were embedded as information in discrete molecules in the same way that genetic information is embedded in DNA, and that these memories were transferable from brain to brain. A later experiment by Baylor University's Georges Ungar was the most vivid yet: Brain cells from rats that had been trained to fear the dark were transferred to untrained mice (ordinarily, neither mice nor rats fear the dark), who suddenly took on this new fear. Ungar even isolated a peptide comprising fifteen amino acids that he said contained the newly created memory. He called the transmissible fear-of-the-dark memory molecule *scotophobin*.

The theory that emerged out of these experiments was of memory as a distinct informational molecule that could be created organically in one brain, isolated, and then transferred to another brain—even to the brain of another species. Its implications were immense. Had this cold fusion of an idea been validated rather than widely discredited not long after Ungar's paper was published in *Nature* in 1972, it is clear that ours would be a very different world today: Memory swaps. Consciousness transfers. Neurochemical behavioral enhancements that would make Prozac seem like baby aspirin. The rapid decoding of a hidden science of memory molecules might well have spawned a new type of biochemical computer that could register, react to, and even *create* memory molecules of its own. Laptops (or cars or stuffed animals) could be afraid of the dark or partial to jazz or concerned about child abuse. Memories and feelings could be bottled and sold as easily as perfume.

But that world did not, and cannot, emerge. The memory transfer experiments, while entertaining and even seductive— DNA pioneer Francis Crick was among the many prestigious scientists on board for a while—were ultimately dismissed as seriously misguided). The idea of transferable memories strained credulity to begin with; to suggest that one animal's specific fear could travel through another animal's digestive tract, enter its bloodstream, find its way to the brain, and turn itself on again in the new host mind was an even further stretch.

And then there was the problem of physical mass. Skeptics calculated that if specific memories were contained in molecules the way Ungar suggested, the total number of memories accumulated over a lifetime would weigh somewhere in the vicinity of 220 pounds. The brain would literally be weighed down by thought and ideas.

After a decade or so, the notion and burgeoning industry of memory molecules crumbled into dust. It is now one particularly humiliating memory that many neuroscientists would just as soon not retain. What has grown up out of that rubble over the last thirty years is a very different understanding of memory—not as a substance but as a *system*. Memories are scattered about; that part the memory molecularists had right. Memory *is* everywhere. But it is everywhere in such a way that it is impossible to point to any one spot and identify it with an explicit memory. We now know that memory, like consciousness itself, isn't a thing that can be isolated or extracted, but a living process, a vast and dynamic interaction of neuronal synapses involved in what Harvard's Daniel Schacter elegantly terms "a temporary constellation of activity." Each specific memory is a unique network of neurons from different regions of the brain coordinating with one another. Schacter explains:

> A typical incident in our everyday lives consists of numerous sights, sounds, actions, and words. Different areas of the brain analyze these various aspects of an event. As a result, neurons in the different regions become more strongly connected to one another. The new pattern of connections constitutes the brain's record of the event.

The power of the constellation idea is reinforced by the understanding of just how connected the 100 billion neurons in the brain actually are. A. G. Cairns-Smith, of the University of Glasgow, observes that no single brain cell is separated from any other brain cell by more than six or seven intermediaries.

The molecular basis for these synaptic constellations that can be reignited again and again (though never in precisely the same configuration), is a biochemical process called long-term potentiation (LTP) that intensifies the affinity between specific neurons after a significant connection is made. Think of an ant farm, with worker ants constantly building new tunnels among one another; once a tunnel is built, transport becomes many times easier; an easy, natural connection has been created between those two points. With memory formation and retrieval, pathways are at first built and later simply used. Each notable experience causes a unique set of neurons to fire in conjunction with one another. As a result, those connections become chemically more sensitive to one another so that they can more easily trigger each other again. With that unique constellation of synapses, one has created a permanent physical trace of the original sensation. Neurologists call these memory traces "engrams."

The ant farm analogy also applies in another important way: Neurobiologists have found that memory formation is *slow*. Long-term memories can take many months or even years to fully form.

Long-term memories are durable, but not unassailable. They can last a lifetime, but from the first moments are subject to influences from other memories and experience. Inevitably, as they age and are evoked again and again, all memories change in character.

This is part of the brain's famous plasticity, its ability to adapt to life's events. Plasticity makes us as much creatures of our own experience as we are products of evolution. Not everything in the brain is adaptable, of course; much of it comes "hard-wired," genetically preprogrammed to specialize and perform specific tasks such as processing light and sound, regulating heart rate and breathing, and so on. But the regions reserved for fine motor skills, intelligence, and memory are more like soft clay, able to take on a definite shape and yet remain constantly responsive to new stimuli.

Memory constellations, then, are not fixed, immutable collections of memories, but ever-variable collections of memory fragments that come together in the context of a specific conscious moment. Any common free-association experiment is a vivid illustration of this point. For me, at this moment, the word "cat" prompts ⟶ a thought of Brownfoot, my boyhood feline friend ⟶ the garage roof she used to leap from ⟶ the 1971 T-top Corvette my father used to drive ⟶ the tragicomic month in which Mom wrecked this car twice ⟶ a feeling of malaise associated with my parents' divorce years later. This instant montage of memories is neither chronological nor predictable, even by me. If someone were to prompt me with "cat" tomorrow, depending on my mood or recent experience, I might think of the cat that my daughter called to yesterday outside our house. Or it could be that Brownfoot will come to mind, but that from there I will shift to an image of my playing her dentist, and then I might think of my own current dentist and how I'm way overdue for a cleaning. That guilty feeling might then trigger another distant idea, related only by a parallel feeling of guilt. And so on.

Taken together, this interconnected universe of constellations in each of us forms the core of who we are. Our life's ocean full of memory waves wash against one another to create a complex and ever-adapting character.

The director Martin Scorsese is an interesting memory-character study, mostly because he seems to forget very little compared to others. He remembers not just every shot and crew credit from each of the thousands of movies he's seen, observes the *New Yorker*'s Mark Singer, but also every detail of every book, song, and personal experience he's had in fifty-plus years—"all of it," Singer writes, "seemingly instantly retrievable."

Singer depicts the Scorsese memory constellation in action. After a colleague criticizes a piece of film dialogue as "too piercing," Scorsese is instantly thrown into an interconnected memory odyssey:

> He was reminded of the old Harry Belafonte calypso tune "The Banana Boat Song"—or, rather, a parody of same by Stan Freberg, which included a reference to "piercing," and that reminded him of another Freberg routine, a parody of the television series *Dragnet,* which in turn reminded him of *Pete Kelly's Blues,* a feature film directed by Jack Webb, the star of *Dragnet.* The production designer of *Pete Kelly's Blues,* in which Webb played a bandleader during the twenties, was a Disney veteran who brought to it a remarkably vivid palette, a reality-heightening Technicolor glow reminiscent of the live-action Disney children's films of the forties. . . . And, Scorsese further recalled, *Pete Kelly's Blues* had a screenplay by Richard L. Breen, whose name, curiously, Webb had heralded before the title. When the picture was released, in 1955, the year Scorsese turned thirteen, he fol-

lowed it from theatre to theatre, as was his habit. . . . [He then recalled all the specific theaters he used to frequent.] One particular Saturday afternoon double-feature at the Orpheum came to
mind: *Bomba the Jungle Boy* and *Great White Hunter*. . . .

The pathways linking engrams can be built on temporal, intellectual, or aesthetic associations, and when the mind really wan-
ders, during daydreams or at night before sleep sets in, it's amazing
what sort of involuntary memory leaps one makes, from impressions that often have no logical or logistical relationship but which
share a texture or smell or emotional fragment. What's more—and
this may be the single most important point to understand about
memory—*every time a memory is recalled, new trails are made.*

The act of remembering itself generates new memories. Which
means that Emerson was exactly right when he noted in his journal: "Most remembering is only the memory of memories, & not
a new & primary remembrance . . . HDT [Henry David Thoreau]
noticed this to me some time ago." Overlap, in other words, is not
only built into the biology of memory. It is the very basis of memory—and identity. New memory traces are laid down on top of a
foundation of old memories, and old memories can only be recalled in a context of recent experiences. Imagine a single painting
being created over the course of a lifetime on one giant canvas.
Every brush stroke coming into contact with many others can be
seen only in the context of those prior strokes—and also instantly
alters those older strokes. Because of this, no recorded experience
can ever be fully distinct from anything else. Whether one likes it
or not, the past is always informed by the present, and vice versa.

Scores of experiments confirm the malleability of old memories, and horror stories of False Memory Syndrome are by now widespread. The psychologist Elizabeth Loftus has spent the better part of her career documenting the ease with which false memories can be planted—accidentally or on purpose. Often, these false memories lead to wrongful convictions. In 1979, twenty-two-year-old marine corporal Kevin Green was convicted of second-degree murder for the brutal beating of his wife and the death of their full-term fetus. His wife had testified after coming out of a coma that Green, her own husband, was the attacker. Sixteen years later, the real attacker, a total stranger, confessed to police about that and six other murders. It turned out that Green's guilt had been suggested to his wife early on in her rehabilitation. By the time it came to trial, she had created a memory so clear that she was able to confidently testify against her husband.

"Eyewitness misidentification . . . is known as the single greatest cause of the conviction of the innocent," says attorney Barry Scheck. He describes a typical scenario: "You can have as many as five witnesses who begin in kind of a soft way, saying, 'That *might* be the guy,' and then, like wet concrete hardening, the [memories] get fixed to the point that by the time they get to the courtroom, they're saying *'That's* the man.' "

Part of the deep attraction to the idea of distinct memory molecules was that it connoted the ability to *replay* old memories like videotapes on a VCR—just as they were originally recorded. But the biology of memory constellations dictates that there is no such thing as pure memory. *Recall* is never *replay.*

But why? Why would millions of years of evolution produce a machine so otherwise sophisticated but with an apparent built-in fuzziness, a tendency to regularly forget, repress, and distort information and experience?

The answer, it turns out, is that fuzziness is not a severe limitation but a highly advanced feature. As a matter of engineering, the brain does not have any physical limitations in the amount of information it can hold. It is designed specifically to forget most of the details it comes across, so that it may allow us to form general impressions, and from there useful judgments. Forgetting is not a failure at all, but an active metabolic process, a flushing out of data in the pursuit of knowledge and meaning.

We know this not just from brain chemistry and inference, but also because psychologists have stumbled upon a few individuals over the years who actually could not forget *enough*—and were debilitated by it.

In his *New Yorker* profile, Mark Singer wonders if Martin Scorsese is such a person—burdened by too good a memory.

> Was it, I wondered, painful to remember so much? Scorsese's powers of recall weren't limited to summoning plot turns or notable scenes or acting performances; his gray matter bulged with camera angles, lighting strategies, scores, sound effects, ambient noises, editing rhythms, production credits, data about lenses and film stocks and exposure speeds and aspect ratios. . . . What about all the sludge? An inability to forget the forgettable—wasn't that a burden, or was it just part of the price one paid to make great art?

For some perspective on the inability to forget, consider the case study that psychologists call *S.* In the 1920s, *S.* was a twenty-something newspaper reporter in Moscow who one day got into trouble with his editor for not taking notes at a staff meeting. In the midst of the reprimand, S. shocked his boss by matter-of-factly repeating everything that had been said in the meeting—word for word.

This was apparently no stretch at all for S., who, it emerged upon closer examination, remembered virtually every detail of sight and sound that he had come into contact with in his entire life. What's more, he took this perfect memory entirely for granted. To him, it seemed perfectly normal that he forgot nothing.

The editor, amazed, sent S. to the distinguished Russian psychologist A. R. Luria for testing. Luria did test him that day, and for many other days over a period of many decades. In all the testing, he could not find any real limit to his capacity to recall details. For example, not only could he perfectly recall tables like this one full of random data after looking at them for just a few minutes:

6	6	8	0
5	4	3	2
1	6	8	4
7	9	3	5
4	2	3	7
3	8	9	1
1	0	0	2
3	4	5	1
2	7	6	8
1	9	2	6
2	9	6	7
5	5	2	0
x	0	1	x

And not only could he efficiently recite these tables backwards, upside down, diagonally, etc., but after years of memorizing thousands of such tables he could easily reproduce any particular one of them, without warning, whether it was an hour after he had first seen it, or twenty years. The man, it seemed, quite literally remembered everything.

And yet he understood almost nothing. S. was plagued by an inability to make meaning out of what he saw. Unless one pointed the obvious pattern out to him, for example, the following table appeared just as bereft of order and meaning as any other:

1	2	3	4
2	3	4	5
3	4	5	6
4	5	6	7

"If I had been given the letters of the alphabet arranged in a similar order," he remarked after being questioned about the 1–2–3–4 table, "I wouldn't have noticed their arrangement." He was also unable to make sense out of poetry or prose, to understand much about the law, or even to remember people's faces. "They're so changeable," he complained to Luria. "A person's expression depends on his mood and on the circumstances under which you happen to meet him. People's faces are constantly changing; it's the different shades of expression that confuse me and make it so hard to remember faces."

Luria also noted that S. came across as generally disorganized, dull-witted, and without much of a sense of purpose or direction in life. This astounding man, then, was not so much gifted with the ability to remember everything as he was cursed with the inability to forget detail and form more general impressions. He recorded only information, and was bereft of the essential ability to draw meaning out of events. "Many of us are anxious to find ways to improve our memories," wrote Luria in a lengthy report on his unusual subject. "In S.'s case, however, precisely the reverse was true. The big question for him, and the most troublesome, was how he could learn to forget."

What makes details hazy also enables us to prioritize information, recognize and retain patterns. The brain eliminates trees in order to make sense of, and remember, the forests. Forgetting is a hidden virtue. Forgetting is what makes us so smart.

⌀

One of the worst things that I have to do is put on my pants in the morning. This morning I kept thinking there is something wrong because my pants just didn't feel right. I had put them on wrong. I sometimes will have to put them on and take them off half a dozen times or more. . . . Setting the washing machine is getting to be a problem, too. Sometimes I'll spend an hour trying to figure out how to set it.

—B.
San Diego, California

⌀

Chapter 4

THE RACE

❦

Taos

"Ten years to a cure," a Japanese scientist whispered to me in our hotel lobby as we waited for the shuttle bus to the Taos Civic Plaza.

The whisper was as telling as the words. He couldn't contain his optimism, and yet he also couldn't afford to put it on display.

Other Alzheimer's researchers had lately been adopting a similar posture. As scientists, they were reserved by nature. But the recent acceleration of discovery had made them a little giddy. Hundreds of important discoveries had come in recent years, and funding for research was way up. The study of Alzheimer's was now in the top scientific tier, alongside heart disease, cancer, and stroke research. This seemed fitting, since the disease was emerging as one of the largest causes of death in the U.S., not far behind those other three.

There was now even an Alzheimer's drug on the market, Aricept, introduced in 1997, which boosted the brain's supply of the neurotransmitter acetylcholine. Some of the functional loss in early Alzheimer's involves a deficiency of acetylcholine; replenishing it with this drug seemed to help about half of early and middle-stage patients to slow or even arrest the progression of symptoms for a year or more.

On the one hand, this was a giant advance: a real treatment that often made a tangible difference. But it was also a frustrating baby-step: Aricept did *not* slow the advance of the actual disease by a single day. It only worked on the symptoms. Scientists couldn't stop Alzheimer's yet—only put a thick curtain in front of it for a while.

More ambitious advances were brewing. An electronic update service named *Alzheimer's Weekly* had been launched in 1998. Neurologists in the 1960s would have considered this phrase a sarcastic reference to the drudging nature of discovery: Understanding of the disease was practically frozen for more than half a decade. But after a thaw in the 1970s and a renewed effort in the '80s, genetic and molecular discoveries started to cascade so quickly by the mid-1990s that the excavation of Alzheimer's seemed to be moving at the same clip as sporting events and financial markets.

Now a weekly update was not only useful but essential. In fact, updates on other Web sites came almost daily:

News from the Research Front

3 September 1998. H. J. Song et al. report that they are able to manipulate growth cones . . .

5 September 1998. Puny polymer pellets show promise as a vehicle for delivering nerve-growth factor to the basal forebrain . . .

6 September 1998. A novel brain-imaging agent promises to open up a window on the functioning of the brain's dopamine system . . .

10 September 1998. Findings published in *Nature Neuroscience* indicate that the accumulation of calcium in the mitochondria triggers neuronal death . . .

10 September 1998. C. Y. Wang et al. report they have identified four genes that are targets of NF-kB activity . . .

11 September 1998. E. Nedivi et al. describe CPG15, a molecule that enhances dendritic arbor growth in projection neurons . . .

—from the *Alzheimer Research Forum* (at www.alzforum.org)

The research was so intensely specialized that few individual scientists appeared to even be working on the problem of Alzheimer's disease *per se.* It was more like each was unearthing a single two-inch tile in a giant mosaic. By themselves, these individual experiments were so narrowly focused that they were far removed from a comprehensive understanding of the disease. But the minutiae had a purpose. If the great challenge of Alois Alzheimer had been to distinguish a general pathology of dementia from the normal cells of the brain, the task of contemporary scientists—employing exotic techniques with names like fluorescent protein tagging, immuno-lesioning, and western blot analysis—was to try to see what the process looked like in flux. Alzheimer glimpsed a mono-colored, silver-stained microscopic snapshot. Contemporary scientists, crunching and exchanging data with parallel processors and fiber optics, were trying to patch together more of a motion picture. Once they understood the actual disease *process,* particularly the early molecular events, they hoped they would be able to proceed toward genuine therapies.

The research had expanded in every direction, and had also gone global. Thousands of scientists from every continent now worked on the problem, as time became critical. In a little over a decade, the much-anticipated "senior boom" would begin, eventually quadrupling the number of Alzheimer's cases and making it the fastest-growing disease in developed countries. In addition to the sheer misery, the social costs of such a slow, progressive disease would be staggering. In the U.S., the costs of doctor's visits, lab tests, medicine, nursing, day care, and home care was already estimated to be $114.4 billion annually. That was more than the combined budgets for the U.S. Departments of Commerce, Education, Energy, Justice, Labor, and Interior.

"We have to solve this problem, or it's going to overwhelm us," Zaven Khachaturian said. "The numbers are going to double every twenty years. Not only that: The duration of illness is going to get much longer. That's the really devastating part. The folks who have the disease now are mostly people who came through the Depression. Some had college education, but most did not. The ones who are going to develop Alzheimer's in the next century will be baby boomers who are primarily much better educated and better fed. The duration of their disability is going to be much longer than the current crop. That's going to be a major factor.

"See, in considering the social impact of the disease, it's not so much the pain and suffering that matters. From the point of view of the individual, that is of course the important factor. But from the point of view of society, what's important is how long I am disabled and how much of a burden I am to society. With cancer and heart disease, the period where I cannot function independently is fairly short—three to five years. With Alzheimer's, it's going to be extremely long—like twenty years, where you are physically there, you don't have any pain, you appear normal, and yet you have Alzheimer's. You *cannot* function independently."

If Khachaturian was correct, and the average duration of the disease was set to more than double, then the problem would be even worse than epidemiologists were predicting. Either way, it was clear that if Alzheimer's disease was not conquered reasonably soon, it would become one of the most prominent features of our future. Nationally, the number of nursing home beds would at least quadruple. (The stay of Alzheimer's sufferers in a nursing home is, on average, twice as long as that of other patients.) We would need vastly more home health care workers, elder-care nurses and physicians, assisted living facilities, day-care programs and support groups. (There was already a grave shortage of qualified professional caregivers—and, due to the low pay, a shocking annual turnover rate of 94 percent.) Family leave would also have to be redefined. Progressive nations would likely adopt a system of employee flexibility for senior care (extended leave, flexible work hours, and so on) similar to the one recently implemented for new parents in the U.S.—with the added caveat that *reverse parenthood* lasts significantly longer and is more draining than conventional parenthood.

All this would cost money, and would require a painful shift in resources away from other public needs. Public officials would be forced into difficult decisions. Would the U.S. government, for example, continue to allow an Alzheimer's patient to give away all assets to his children in order to qualify for government-sponsored care? Would governments require citizens to have some sort of dementia or frailty insurance?

And what about public safety issues? With as many as fifteen million people suffering from insidious (and largely invisible) cognitive decline, how would we insure street and highway safety without automatically invalidating all driver's licenses of senior citizens?

There was a dual race on, then. Researchers were racing against one another, and against time. The prize for the winner of this race—if there was to be a winner—would be worldwide fame, nearly unparalleled professional esteem, enormous wealth, and the pride of knowing that you were personally responsible for preventing an ocean of future human suffering.

One glimpse into the magnitude of an Alzheimer's cure: In the nearly fifty years since Jonas Salk and Albert Sabin introduced their vaccines against polio, somewhere between 1 and 2 million lives have been saved. Curing Alzheimer's disease sometime in the first decade of the twenty-first century would save as many as 100 million lives worldwide in the same length of time.

The far-flung researchers kept in touch by E-mail, phone, and fax, and accomplished much in their labs spread out all over the world. Still, every so often, they needed to come together physically, to be in the same room to check their progress, to goad each other, critique and criticize each other, to energize.

In 1999, the gathering place was Taos. They came from everywhere, a global convergence of neuromolecular intelligentsia sitting on fold-out chairs in Bataan Hall to share knowledge and probe their ignorance. There was still so much they didn't know: Why are women more susceptible to Alzheimer's than men? Why are Cree and Cherokee Indians less susceptible than the rest of us? What is it about the environment in Hawaii, as contrasted with Japan, that apparently doubles one's chances of getting Alzheimer's? Why do a third of Alzheimer's victims develop Parkinson's disease but not the other two-thirds? Why do some cigarette smokers seem to be *less* likely to develop Alzheimer's than nonsmokers?

After ninety-plus years, the field was littered with half-answers to these questions—and far more basic ones: Does Alzheimer's have one cause or many? Is it really one disease or a collection of very similar diseases? Which come first—plaques or tangles? Why do they always originate in the same part of the brain? How long do they proliferate before they begin to affect brain performance? Why do some people accrue a brain full of plaques and tangles but never display any symptoms of the disease? Is anyone naturally immune to Alzheimer's?

So, humbly, they gathered. With respect for the vexing nature of this disease, the molecular biologists and geneticists spent thirty hours listening to theories of plaque and tangle formation, and intervention strategies. After each short talk, they quickly lined up behind a microphone in the aisle to poke the presenter with questions, looking for holes in the research and analysis. The tone was alternately respectful and suspicious, and occasionally hostile.

Hostile because of the billions of dollars at stake, and also because of a fracturing debate within the community about which aspect of research mattered most. A nearly one-hundred-year-old question still had not been answered: Which are closer to the root of the problem—the plaques or the tangles?

Alois Alzheimer thought it was the tangles. "We have to con-

clude," he wrote in 1911, "that the plaques are not the cause of senile dementia but only an accompanying feature."

Most, however, now said the plaques. In a field where there
were so many open questions and possible approaches, the vast
majority of researchers in this room and elsewhere were focused
tightly on the issue of plaque formation, while relatively few were
concerned with tangles and only a handful of others busied themselves with important issues like inflammation, viruses, and possible environmental factors.

The disparity bothered many. "When I was a little girl, I
wanted to go into science because I thought it was a very open
community," Ruth Itzhaki, a biologist from the University of
Manchester, told me one morning in Taos. "I learned better. It is,
in fact, a very cynical community layered with politics and filled
with people who just want to follow the herd." Itzhaki was herself
embittered by her struggle to fund research linking the herpes simplex virus 1 (HSV1) with Alzheimer's.

Could Alzheimer's be herpes of the brain? It was not the most
prominent theory of the day, but no one could rule it out. Nearly
all humans are infected by HSV1 by the time they reach middle
age. The virus mostly seems to lie dormant but can become active
and create cold sores and other hazards in times of stress. Whether
or not HSV1 does any damage depends largely on individual levels of immune response and on genetic makeup.

In her presentation, Itzhaki said she had found evidence of
HSV1 presence in the temporal and frontal cortex of the brain, as
well as in the hippocampus—three areas closely associated with
Alzheimer's. She posited that the virus might be interacting with a
particular gene to set the disease process in motion. If proven true,

a massive new global infant immunization project would be in order.

But the crowd in Taos did not seem very interested. Her talk drew little in the way of response. The focus quickly shifted back to plaques.

One evening I got a telephone call from a friend. He was telling me what a tough day he'd had on the job; he'd made several mistakes. "If you have Alzheimer's, I must have a double dose of it," he said.

I could feel myself entering a state of rage. "Do you forget simple words, or substitute inappropriate words, making your sentences incomprehensible? Do you cook a meal and not only forget you cooked it, but forget to eat it? Do you put your frying pan in the freezer, or your wallet in the sugar bowl, only to find them later and wonder what in the world is happening to you? Do you become lost on your own street? Do you mow your lawn three or four times a day? When you balance your checkbook, do you completely forget what the numbers are and what needs to be done with them? Do you become confused or fearful ten times a day, for no reason? And most of all, do you become irate when someone makes a dumb statement like you just made?"

"No."

"Then you don't have Alzheimer's," I said, and hung up.

—L.R.
Lafayette, Louisiana

Chapter 5

IRRESPECTIVE OF AGE

⌒

Late one night in the early 1950s, Meta Neumann, a neuropathologist at St. Elizabeth's Hospital in Washington, D.C., got word that an elderly colleague of hers, the clinical psychiatrist Dr. P., had died. It came without warning. That very morning, Dr. P. had ably led a vigorous meeting of hospital staff.

Situated on a three-hundred-acre campus across the Anacostia River in the southeast quadrant of the District, St. Elizabeth's was at the time the premier mental hospital in the United States. It had been founded a century earlier, in 1855, the first national mental health facility, as part of a massive effort throughout the Western world to rehabilitate the mentally ill. By the mid-twentieth century, St. Elizabeth's housed between seven and eight thousand patients. The poet Ezra Pound was confined there from 1946 to 1958 for his pro-Fascist broadcasts from Italy during World War II. In 1981, it became the home of John Hinckley, Jr., Ronald Reagan's would-be assassin.

St. Elizabeth's also had the oldest pathology lab of any mental health institution, including an unmatched archive of twenty-three hundred brains taken from deceased residents. These preserved brains floated in formaldehyde inside large clear glass jars. For more than a decade, Neumann had been the curator of the brain bank, regularly adding specimens to it and using it for research.

Now Dr. P.'s brain would become an unexpected addition to the collection. The morning after his sudden death, Neumann performed an autopsy on him. She was a specialist in neurodegenerative disorders, and so it didn't take her long to notice something unsettling about the brain of Dr. P. It was badly sclerotic. The arteries in his brain were severely clogged with fatty deposits, much like heart vessels before a major heart attack.

In itself, the cerebral arteriosclerosis was not unusual; indeed, Dr. P. had a classic case. What made it curious was that prior to his death he had not exhibited any of the symptoms of senile dementia. At the time, the medical establishment believed senile dementia—dementia in old age—was caused by cerebral arteriosclerosis, the slow buildup of fat in the brain's arteries over time. Medical schools in the early and mid-twentieth century taught as gospel that there were two clearly distinct types of dementia, easily separated by the age of onset:

Alzheimer's disease—
A very rare disease afflicting people in their forties and fifties, characterized by plaques and tangles. Cause unknown.

Senile dementia—
A relatively common condition affecting the elderly (sixties and older), caused by cerebral arteriosclerosis.

Senile dementia was not regarded as a disease, just an unfortunate side effect of getting old. Few had questioned this distinction, but in Meta Neumann's autopsy lab on that particular morning in 1952, it didn't hold up. According to what she saw in his brain, Dr. P. should have died in a senile fog. But Neumann and her husband, Robert Cohn—also a neuropathologist at St. Elizabeth's (they had met during an autopsy)—had spoken with Dr. P. just before his death, and found him to be perfectly lucid.

If Dr. P. had fatty deposits in his brain, and he wasn't senile, logic dictated that fatty deposits must not cause senility. So, Neumann wondered, what does?

It was a question she could seriously explore on her own. With her own in-house brain bank, she had all the resources she needed at her disposal to examine a large number of cases of diagnosed senile dementia and see if the brains did, in fact, show sclerotic changes. She and Cohn began the hard digging.

Two hundred and ten brains later, her hunch was confirmed. Just as Neumann had suspected, few of the dementia brains showed sclerosis. Instead, they showed plaques and tangles. These were *Alzheimer's* brains.

Alzheimer's was not a rare disease after all. It was the leading cause of dementia, by far, in people of all ages. "The clinical picture was the same," says Cohn, "irrespective of age."

The question of what Alzheimer's disease was, exactly, had been a great sad muddle for many decades, ever since Alois Alzheimer first shared details of his remarkable five-year interaction with Auguste D. as both patient and lab specimen. If the case of Frau D. was destined to be an important part of the history of neuroscience, it was impossible to tell by the initial hearing. Alzheimer discussed his findings at a regional conference for German psychiatrists in November 1906, where he was met with indifference. At the lecture's conclusion, conference chairman Alfred Hoche, a leading psychiatrist from Freiburg, called for questions or comments. No one spoke a word. After a long silence, Hoche called again for questions. Again, nothing. Dementia, death, plaques, tangles—no one in the room seemed to much care. Hoche himself couldn't even muster a comment as a courtesy. "So then, respected colleague Alzheimer, I thank you for your remarks," Hoche said finally. "Clearly there is no desire for discussion."

But the following year, Alzheimer's written report of the autopsy, "A Peculiar Disease of the Cerebral Cortex," was published to a more enthusiastic audience: his boss, Emil Kraepelin.

Kraepelin was the most ambitious and authoritative psychiatrist of the day. In his *Handbook of Psychiatry,* he published the first psychiatric nosology, or classification of diseases. By the early 1890s, it had become an international bestseller, a seminal text. Kraepelin published new editions every few years, and his colleagues regarded his updates and modifications with close attention. By the time of Auguste D.'s death in 1906, Kraepelin was nearly unrivaled in his influence, and not shy about using it.

But Kraepelin was also a man in need. The radical contention of his *Handbook* was that a vast number of mental illnesses were actually organic diseases, with distinct pathologies. The trouble was, he had no proof—no recorded link between mental distress and the alteration of brain tissue. With no evidence to back up his claim, many of Kraepelin's peers loudly doubted his central notion, arguing that brain diseases would never be so easily classifiable from the study of structural changes in the brain. At a 1906 conference in Munich, three prominent psychiatrists confronted him. "There can be no talk of nosological specificity," insisted the distinguished Berlin academic Karl Bonhoeffer.

Robert Gaupp, the new director of the University Hospital for Psychiatry and Psychotherapy in Tübingen, agreed, stating unequivocally, "No psychological symptoms can be explained from anatomical findings."

Alfred Hoche twisted the knife a bit further, poking fun at Kraepelin for what he saw as foolishness. "The search for illness types is a hopeless hunt for a phantom!" teased Hoche.

Only Kraepelin's protégé Alois Alzheimer came to his defense. He did so not only out of loyalty, but also because he had the perfect ammunition. "I can *verify* [this] anatomical doctrine," Alzheimer told the critics flatly. "Twelve days ago, on April 8, a Frankfurt patient, Auguste D., died. I have had the clinical history and the brain sent to Munich, and I have undertaken to document in this case that there is indeed an anatomical doctrine."

Kraepelin's most formidable rival, Viennese neurologist Sigmund Freud, was not at the Munich conference. Freud was fashioning the new school of psychoanalysis out of the proposition that an enormous number of mental problems were neuroses of the mind, not organic diseases of the brain. Where Kraepelin saw the brain as a cell-based organ at the mercy of biological processes, internal mishaps caused by what he called "autotoxins," Freud saw it as a reservoir of thoughts and emotions that played off against one another and competed for dominance. Further, Freud insisted that mental health was not a simple matter of healthy vs. diseased, but more of a continuum. He saw no clear line of demarcation between emotionally healthy and emotionally sick persons.

These competing views would eventually come to be embraced as dually legitimate and coexistent, but in the first decade of the twentieth century, Kraepelin's organic psychiatry and Freud's psychoanalysis were a pair of sumo wrestlers on a small bamboo raft: two ideologies aggressively competing for the same hearts and minds of Central Europe. Co-existence was not considered acceptable to either side.

Kraepelin wrote scathingly of Freud as early as 1899, sarcastically calling his ideas "highly remarkable conceptions" and dismissing what he and his colleagues saw as an obsession with sex. "If . . . our much-plagued soul can lose its equilibrium for all time as a result of long-forgotten unpleasant sexual experiences," Kraepelin remarked, "that would be the beginning of the end of the human race." To the organic psychiatrists standing with Kraepelin, Freud's ideas were little more than *Schweinerei*—"smut." In 1906, Walther Spielmeyer, one of Kraepelin's colleagues, called Freud's work "mental masturbation."

Freud responded with equal acidity. When Otto Gross, one of Kraepelin's clinical assistants, wrote a book that attempted to synthesize both sides of the debate, Freud commented, "What interests me most about Gross's book is that it comes from the clinic of the Super-Pope, or at least was published with his permission."

The critically important brain physiology vs. psychology debate was really just beginning, and would last through the twentieth century and beyond. Along the way, Alzheimer made a significant contribution. As both the physician at Auguste D.'s side and the pathologist examining her brain, Alzheimer established a direct link between her dementia and the plaques and tangles clouding her cortex. This wasn't irrefutable *proof* of an organic brain disease, but it was the first solid evidence. "Alzheimer . . .

offered a causal relation between neuropathological and psychopathological alterations," says psychiatrist and historian Matthias M. Weber. ". . . For this reason, Alois Alzheimer was perhaps the most important coworker of Emil Kraepelin."

After Kraepelin read Alzheimer's article, he immediately seized on the detailed descriptions and moved quickly to formalize the discovery. Grateful to Alzheimer for bolstering his organic doctrine, he probably also wanted to reward him. So he named the disease after him. In the 1910 edition of his *Handbook,* Kraepelin mentioned Alzheimer and his work numerous times before blurting out a surprising and indistinct reference to *Morbus Alzheimer:*

"The clinical interpretation of this Alzheimer's disease is still confused."

Alzheimer's disease was born.

Every disease needs a name. As a matter of social reality, no disease exists until it has one.

Acquired Immunodeficiency Syndrome • Acrocephalosyndactylia • Adams-Stokes Disease • Bell's Palsy • Beriberi • Bloom Syndrome • Blue Rubber Bleb Nevus Syndrome • Bronchitis • Bronchopulmonary Dysplasia • Canavan Disease • Candidiasis • Cherubism • Chicken Pox • Cholangitis • Depression • Dermatofibroma • Dyslexia • Epilepsy • Erb's Palsy • Esotropia • Evans Syndrome • Fibromyalgia • Fuchs' Endothelial Dystrophy • Furunculosis • Giardiasis • Gilbert Disease • Glycogen Storage Disease • Gonorrhea • Goodpasture Syndrome • Hashimoto's Disease • Hematospermia • Hemophilia A • Herpes Simplex • Influenza • Irritable Bowel Syndrome •

Isaac's Syndrome • Job's Syndrome • Keratosis Follicularis • Klinefelter's Syndrome • Klippel-Feil Syndrome • Kuru • Labyrinth Diseases • Laurence-Moon Syndrome • Lemierre's Syndrome • Lentigo • Leukemia • Lyme Disease • Malaria • Malignant Hyperthermia • Measles • Moyamoya Disease • Multiple Myeloma • Multiple Sclerosis • Noonan Syndrome • Nystagmus • Obesity • Oculomotor Nerve Diseases • Osteoarthritis • Pellagra • Pertussis • Pleurisy • Pneumonia • Poland Syndrome • Proctitis • Q Fever • De Quervain's Tendinitis • Reye's Syndrome • Rhabdoid Tumor • Rhinitis • Rocky Mountain Spotted Fever • Romano-Ward Syndrome • Rubella • Sarcoma • Scabies • Scarlet Fever • Scheie Syndrome • Sezary Syndrome • Smallpox • Sprengel's Deformity • Supraglottitis • Syringomyelia • Takayasu's Arteritis • Tay-Sachs Disease • Tinea • Toxic Shock Syndrome • Trichinosis • Typhoid • Undulant Fever • Vasculitis • Volvulus • West Syndrome • Von Willebrand Disease • Wilms' Tumor • Xerostomia • Yaws • Yellow Fever • Zoonoses • Zygomycosis

The disease name is public recognition of a shared affliction. The name says, *THIS is what you are suffering from. You are not alone. Others are suffering from the same thing.*

The name also says, *We're going to fight this thing.* "Choosing to call a set of phenomena a disease," writes medical philosopher H. Tristram Engelhardt, Jr., "involves a commitment to medical intervention, the assignment of the sick-role, and the enlistment in action of health professionals." Naming a disease is tantamount to launching an assault against that disease.

Finally, the name is also a necessary tag for an otherwise intangible phenomenon. A disease is not a *thing* but a *process;* it is neither the cause of the problem nor its visible effects—neither the virus infecting the tissue nor the damaged tissue itself—but the interaction between the two. Because of the elusive nature of disease, the name is often the only available emblem. Once accepted, specific names quickly come to dominate social reality. The flavor of the name can make a real difference in how the disease is perceived and acted on.

Any casual observer can easily see that the history of disease-naming is a haphazard one, four thousand years of jigs and jags that have left us with appellations ranging from the vaguely mythological ("influenza" originally referred to the vast influence of the gods) to the icily clinical (acquired immunodeficiency syndrome). A disease might be named after the major symptom (smallpox), a side effect (yellow fever), a known or suspected cause (schistosomiasis, tuberculosis), or might instead be a vague reference to a social consequence (the plague).

The sporadic tradition of naming a disease after the identifying physician seems to have started in the mid-nineteenth century, when French neurologist Jean-Martin Charcot coined the name *"la maladie de Parkinson"* after London physician James Parkinson's 1817 "Essay on the Shaking Palsy." Thomas Addison earned the honor of "Addison's disease" in 1855 by characterizing a complex disorder involving the destruction of the adrenal glands. Huntington's disease is named after George Huntington, who in 1872 detailed the hereditary chorea that begins with muscle spasms and ends in dementia.

Kraepelin followed in this nascent tradition by naming what seemed to be a new discovery after the discoverer. It was also a political maneuver with two obvious payoffs for the namer. By bringing attention to this new disease, he ensured the maximum possible exposure for the emerging evidence of organic brain disease. And in fashioning a formal new disease after a staff member, Kraepelin also gained additional glory for his own institute.

But what was the disease, exactly? Kraepelin wrote:

> The clinical interpretation of this Alzheimer's disease is still confused. While the anatomical findings suggest that we are dealing with a particularly serious form of senile dementia, the fact that this disease sometimes starts already around the age of fifty does not allow this supposition. In such cases we should at least presume a "senium praecox" [premature aging] if not perhaps a more or less age-independent unique disease process.

The words dropped onto the medical community like a giant crop circle—it was a powerful, resonant event, but what exactly did it mean? Even as the term "Alzheimer's disease" quickly gained currency throughout the world, largely on the strength of Kraepelin's formidable reputation (he would eventually come to be known as the "Linnaeus of psychiatry" for his importance in mental disease classification), it confused many.

On the one hand, it seemed that he intended Alzheimer's disease to refer only to a rare form of so-called presenile dementia that affected a tiny number of people in their forties and fifties. On the other hand, he included his description in the "senile dementia" section of his book, not the presenile section. Also, his suggestion that this was "perhaps a more or less age-independent unique disease process" seemed to imply that the disease could affect anyone, irrespective of age.

Kraepelin's suggestion was strangely jumbled for a man whose life's work had been orderly classification. In one short sentence, he somehow managed both to brazenly introduce a new disease and to undermine it.

On the surface, it seemed like sloppiness. But it could not have been. Kraepelin wasn't blind to the ricochet effect of his words. Far from it: he was as much a political animal as a medical man, running the highest-profile psychiatric clinic in Germany (and arguably in all of Europe). Nor was he known for carelessness. Medical scholars looking back over the span of a century to particulars of his work are continually impressed with his precision and intelligence.

He did it on purpose, as a way of recognizing Alois Alzheimer's genuine discovery but sidestepping the question of how it challenged thousands of years of thinking about old age. For whatever reason, Kraepelin did not want to be the one to suddenly insist that senility was a disease to be fought. "Accepting Alzheimer's disease as a separate disease prevented the coming about of another, more complicated question, i.e., the question whether senile dementia is a disease entity to be distinguished from aging," suggests Dutch physician and historian Rob Dillman.

So Kraepelin left it as "perhaps."

He left it fuzzy, proposing Alzheimer's as a middle-age dementia—and "perhaps" a senile dementia.

Still, it was the first strong hint that senility was not a reasonable part of aging. For all of human history, senile dementia had been tacitly accepted as merely a lamentable stage of life. "But if I am to live on," the Greek historian Xenophon wrote in *Memorabilia* (fourth century B.C.), "haply [by chance] I may be forced to pay the old man's forfeit—to become sand-blind and deaf and dull of wit, slower to learn, quicker to forget, outstripped now by those who were behind me."

In Ecclesiasticus 3.12–13 (second century B.C.) we find these words: "O son, help your father in his old age, and do not grieve him as long as he lives/even if he is lacking in understanding, show forbearance."

Most prominently of all, Shakespeare defined senility as one of life's natural stages. In *As You Like It*, Jaques declares:

. . . one man in his time plays many parts. . . .
Last scene of all,
That ends this strange eventful history,
Is second childishness and mere oblivion. . . .

Even as recently as Ralph Waldo Emerson's steady sinking into what a biographer called his "soft oblivion," through the 1870s and up to his death in 1882, his condition was lamented but accepted with an unwavering fatalism. This isn't particularly surprising, given that in his own notebook Emerson had noted his admiration for a remark by his friend Bronson Alcott on the subject of senility: "That as the child loses, as he comes into the world, his angelic memory, so the man, as he grows old, loses his memory of this world."

The voluminous records of Emerson's life suggest that he saw a doctor about his failing memory only once; apparently, nothing noteworthy came from it. And Edward Emerson, a physician, made no medical observations of his father's condition. Though the disorder attacked Emerson's single greatest asset, his mind, there was no public or private suggestion of *treating* his memory loss, *fighting* it, or in any way considering it a disease. Indeed, when a friend inquired about Emerson's health late in his life, he replied, "Quite well; I have lost my mental faculties but am perfectly well." It is striking to see, through the prism of modern medicine, the stark separation of Emerson's senility from his physical health.

Now, less than three decades after Emerson's ordeal, Kraepelin was suggesting that *perhaps* senile dementia was not just a matter of aging or accelerated aging. *Perhaps* it was a disease; *perhaps* doctors now had a moral obligation to do something about it.

Years passed and the world forgot about Kraepelin's "perhaps." Alzheimer's disease congealed in medical circles as a rare, middle-aged disorder. It came to Meta Neumann and Robert Cohn in 1953 to challenge that thinking with new and convincing evidence. "There is no difference in the clinical or pathological picture in the various age groups," they wrote in their article, published that year in the *Archives of Neurology and Psychiatry.*

The data were meticulous and compelling, but not nearly enough to force a change in convention. Proof or no proof, people weren't ready to call senility a disease. "They didn't believe it," Cohn recalled of colleagues' reactions to the paper they published. "They felt that Meta was talking nonsense."

In the eyes of the psychiatric community, "Alzheimer's" remained a designation for a very rare presenile disease. Senility remained a natural part of aging.

The confusion endured.

A.P.: *On the kitchen door, I have little yellow*
Post-it Notes. So when I leave the house I know I
have to do certain things. I can't go out until I
see that note on the door.

M.W.: *I do the same sort of thing, except that I have a*
big calendar in my kitchen.

T.R.: *I have a book I write in every day.*

J.J.: *Well, I make a list in the kitchen and then one*
in the bedroom. They are the same.
Sometimes in the bathroom I put a different list.

H.K.: *I never thought of that. That sounds so good, to*
have two lists—one on one end of the house and
another on the other end—
because by the time I get back to the other end I
think, "Why have I come?"

—*Houston, Texas*

Chapter 6

A MOST LOVING BROTHER

~Q·

In 75 A.D., Plutarch chronicled the exuberant life and gloomy decline of the great Roman warrior-diplomat Lucius Licinius Lucullus, who fought in Italy and Asia under the emperor Sulla and subsequently governed Africa. After retiring to a life of extravagance, he slid into full-blown dementia. Lucullus's intellect, said Plutarch, "failed him by degrees . . . so disabled and unsettled his mind, that while he was yet alive, his brother took charge of his affairs."

Of the ordeal, Plutarch seemed most impressed by the burden cast on Lucullus's brother Marcus. It was Marcus who had to manage Lucullus's slow decline, as well as his estate. And when Lucullus died (at age fifty-three), it was Marcus who stood up to popular pressure to bury the body in the Field of Mars alongside Sulla. Marcus instead honored Lucullus's specific request that he be buried on his own family grounds. A short time later, Marcus himself was buried in the same spot, no doubt worn down by his tireless duties in service to his ailing brother. Admiring Marcus's sacrifice, Plutarch closed his long essay with a benediction not for the famous victim but his caregiver. "In all respects," he wrote, "a most loving brother."

The unique curse of Alzheimer's is that it ravages several victims for every brain it infects. Since it shuts down the brain very slowly, beginning with higher functions, close friends and loved ones are forced not only to witness an excruciating fade but also increasingly to step in and compensate for lost abilities. We all rely on the assistance of other people in order to live full, rich lives. A person with dementia relies increasingly—and, in the fullness of time, *completely*—on the care of others. Lucullus had his brother. Reagan has his wife and Secret Service agents. Greta, Arnie, and Doris have their doctors, nurses, spouses, siblings, children, and friends.

The caregiver must preside over the degeneration of someone he or she loves very much; must do this for years and years with the news always getting worse, not better; must every few months learn to compensate for new shortcomings with makeshift remedies; must negotiate impossible requests and fantastic observations; must put up sometimes with deranged but at the same time very personal insults; and must somehow learn to smile through it all. The work shift in this literally thankless job lasts for twenty-four hours a day, seven days a week. On-the-job training includes basic neurology, nursing 101, and mind reading. Caregivers must be able to diagnose a wide variety of ordinary ailments—toothache, nausea, urinary tract infection, and so on—under extraordinary circumstances. Imagine a patient suddenly upset about something but completely unable to communicate the problem, or even to understand it himself. Is he hungry? Exhausted? Sore? Does he have a bad headache or did he break his toe? Is his back in spasms or is his appendix inflamed? Can he point to the problem? No, he cannot.

The stress facing caregivers is so extraordinary that it commonly leads to very serious problems on its own. "Caregiver's dementia" is widely used to describe the overpowering symptoms of fatigue and forgetfulness that often come with the role of Alzheimer's caregiver—staying up all hours, going days or weeks without a break, and so on. The term is half tongue in cheek, not intended to refer to a biological dementia. Still, this stress-induced psychological condition can be very, very serious. One estimate has roughly half of all Alzheimer's caregivers struggling with clinical depression.

In the late 1990s, some 10–15 million Americans were called to duty. More often than not they were women, often in their forties or early fifties, often recently retired from the more conventional parenting role after nearly two decades. The kids had just gone off to work or started college; life was supposed to begin all over again—and then a call came in: Mom or Dad had been acting a little strange lately.

There are no wages for this grueling job, of course, and depending on the patient's health insurance and the size of her estate, the illness can actually cost the caregiver tens of thousands of dollars every year. Neither Medicare nor private health insurance covers the type of long-term care most patients need. The average out-of-pocket costs for Alzheimer's patients are $12,500 per year. Nursing home care averages more than $40,000 annually.

If estranged family members don't happen to be sensitive to the burdens of Alzheimer's disease, there might also be substantial legal bills. The very slow fade of a parent often tends to knock pegs out from under already shaky families. In Shakespeare's rendition of *King Lear*, written in 1605–1606, Lear's two elder daughters take cruel advantage of their father's weakening state of mind while the third daughter, Cordelia, suffers for her loyalty and lack of guile. The play is about a family's dissolution through misunderstanding and distrust. Senility is the playwright's device.

It was a striking plot choice. There had been at least fifty versions of the Lear (or "Leir") story prior to Shakespeare's, but his was the first to put the king in a deep senile fog. Throughout Shakespeare's play, Lear hallucinates, doesn't recognize old friends, and cannot remember who he is. "My wits begin to turn," he remarks in one scene; in another, "I am cut to the brains." With a few exceptions (most notably his plot-driven mental recovery in the last act), his complaints are perfectly in synch with the Alzheimer's experience:

> I fear I am not in my perfect mind.
> Methinks I should know you, and know this man;
> Yet I am doubtful; for I am mainly ignorant
> What place this is; and all the skill I have
> Remembers not these garments; nor I know not
> Where I did lodge last night. . . .
>
> —KING LEAR, ACT IV, SCENE 3

Shakespeare's decision to incorporate dementia may have been inspired by the real-life case of Bryan Annesley, a wealthy palace attendant to Shakespeare's patron, Queen Elizabeth. In 1603—two years before Shakespeare wrote *King Lear*—Annesley's senility became a public spectacle in the English court. Annesley was in the late stages of progressive dementia: "Fallen into such imperfection and distemperature of mind and memory," reported an observer, "[and] altogether unfit to govern himself." His youngest daughter (of three), named Cordell, the only one not yet married, remained at home to care for him. By contrast, the eldest daughter, Grace, kept her attentions focused on the sizable estate, suing to have her father declared a lunatic so she could take immediate custody of his possessions.

Under the law at that time, a lunatic was deprived of all civil and human rights and was subject to the whims of the family property owner. Cordell's successful defense of her father's rights— she convinced the royal minister Lord Cecil to place the estate into the custody of a loyal family friend—very likely insured that he would have the most comfortable and dignified descent possible. Annesley died the next year, still under Cordell's care.

Four centuries later, Cordell Annesleys could be found in every city of the world. "My sister-in-law visited for a few days while my mother-in-law was in the hospital," reported Sally D., from Logansport, Indiana. "When I went over to mow the lawn, I found she had rearranged the china cabinet. A lot of stuff was not there. I suppose we should take an inventory of everything in the house, so when the time comes, we can see what has walked away during the interim. We should not have to do this."

Longer lives and the proliferation of Alzheimer's were colliding with yet another modern circumstance—the scattering of families. As if there were not enough layers of sadness already, the disease too often also became a wedge, driving already fractured families further apart. "Things are going from bad to worse here," said Jean B. from Lexington, Massachusetts. "I just got a letter from my sister's law firm about the estate and having to inventory everything in this house. First, they said everything here is Dad's, conveniently ignoring the fact that Ashley and I brought things here and have acquired things subsequently. It also said I was 'staying with' Dad—which has a far different connotation than 'taking care of' Dad—like I am here mooching off him because of some deficiency in my own life."

Though they lived a thousand miles apart, Sally and Jean were able to find and support each other, and hundreds of other caregivers scattered throughout the world, via the Alzheimer List, on the Internet at http://www.adrc.wustl.edu/alzheimer. A virtual support group created by the Alzheimer's Disease Research Center at Washington University in St. Louis in 1994, the list helped more than a thousand caregivers, social workers, clinicians, and researchers form a community through E-mail dispatches. Discussions ranged from whether/how to tell already demented loved ones about their disease, to appropriate dosage levels of medications, to which air fresheners best remove the smell of human feces from a room. For pixels on a screen, the talk was surprisingly warm and intimate.

13 Aug 2000
From: Carla Flaherty
Subject: Visiting Dad at Primrose

Thank you Kathy, Geri, Michelle, Eveline, and Connie for your responses to my sad visits with Dad. You are all, as always, a great help and gave me good thoughts—which made Friday's visit much easier on me.

Yes—two of you mentioned this—what I REALLY want is for Dad to come back for a minute and say, "Hey, you did good, kiddo. I know you didn't want this, and I didn't either, but you did the best you could and I'm satisfied with it." Getting clear that I wanted the impossible made it easier. So I will tell myself these things instead. And pick pears for Dad, knowing I HAVE done the best I could.

Luck & hope,
Carla

Perhaps the Internet was the perfect medium for Alzheimer's caregivers: millions of them sprinkled across the earth, stuck in their homes taking care of their loved ones, rarely able to break away. Then, with little warning, a free moment popped up in the early afternoon or the middle of the night. Down the stairs in a cluttered basement office, a screen and keyboard provided the connection to countless others with similar concerns.

At 2:30 A.M., Diane wrote in from San Diego with a question about her mother's sleeplessness. At 9:00 A.M., a response came from Jerry in Spokane. He patiently recalled his own experience with "sundowning," passing on the array of tactics and tools used, and assuring her that the night restlessness would eventually pass.

Nina from Adrian, Michigan, needed some advice on how to handle her mother's stubborn refusal to allow a nurse into the home. Geri from Minneapolis piped in: She had been through exactly the same thing with her husband, and explained the legal Catch-22: If Nina's mother was already so impaired that she couldn't take care of herself, she was probably also too impaired to give Nina legal authority to make key decisions on her behalf. If so, Nina would have to ask a judge to declare her mother incompetent (the modern equivalent of the Elizabethan "lunatic").

Focused exchanges like this continued twenty-four hours a day, in a never-ending swap of empathy, camaraderie, and advice. After several years and some 14 million words, the group had covered a lot of ground: room monitors, mini-strokes, drug trials, spending sprees, wandering, day care, power of attorney, stages of grieving, assisted living, door knob covers, incontinence, corporate insensitivity, family reunions, caregiver's depression, sadness, terror, relief, betrayal, even attempted murder. Hanging over all the painful details like a wide porch roof was a rich poignancy, a sense that these family members had been tested and dredged for all their depth of feeling. Here were people in the throes of a slow, horrible loss, aggravating and draining, and yet many seemed to be experiencing the fullness of life in a way that made me as a distant observer feel perversely envious. No one in this group seemed dead to the world, stuck in old habits, numb and sleepwalking through daily chores. These people were buzzing with life.

Following their conversations, I realized that while medical science gives us many tools for staying alive, it cannot help us with the art of living—or dying. Life, in its precious transience, is something we can only define on our own terms. With Alzheimer's disease, the caregiver's challenge is to escape the medical confines of *disease* and to assemble a new humanity in the loss.

One realization that popped up over and over again on the List, for example, was the importance of not forcing "reality" onto someone living with Alzheimer's. "During the early years," recalled Rolfe S. from Fairfield, Vermont, "I tried to have Phyllis live life the . . . 'normal' . . . way—my way or our pre-Alzheimer's way of life. It did not work. When I corrected her or tried to 'normalize' her she became agitated, which in turn agitated me and made life hell. She was unhappy. I was unhappy.

"I finally realized that whatever I said or did to correct her made no difference. I realized that life would be easier if I let her do what she wanted (within safety limits). I no longer scolded her but thanked her for bringing the frying pan into the bathroom. After that, life changed very much for the good. She is happy but still declining. I am happy and have adjusted to my new 'life.' It will change some day but if it doesn't, so be it. Enjoy life as best you can."

Over the years, List participants had discussed it all, it seemed. But there were still occasional surprises. In late February 1999, an extraordinary dispatch came in from Morris Friedell, a quiet, bushy-bearded, tweed-coated sociologist from Southern California.

"I first subscribed to this list because of my mother's probable Alzheimer's," Morris wrote. "A neurologist and a neuropsychologist told me my own forgetfulness was probably benign aging plus Caregiver's Dementia. Unfortunately, another neurologist, with the help of an MRI, a PET, and a qEEG, diagnosed me as having Alzheimer's myself."

A patient—on the List? This was something new. The community was well-versed in talking *about* Alzheimer's sufferers, not *to* them.

And that was only half the surprise.

Morris had not come to kvetch. He was no helpless Lear, flailing about, but part of the new class of Alzheimer's sufferers, diagnosed so early as to still be able to speak for themselves, to eloquently describe their experience, and to champion their rights. More than that, even, Morris wanted to talk about *rehabilitation.*

Not long before, this fifty-nine-year-old college professor had been planning his early retirement, hoping to read and write books free from the commitments of teaching. Then memory troubles intervened. During his final year with students, he began to have trouble remembering what his students said in class. Later, he couldn't remember a conversation he'd just had with his mother. At the neuropsychologist's office, he couldn't tell the doctor about a movie he'd seen just the night before. They ran the usual tests. He got a perfect score on the MMSE. On the brain scans, he didn't fare so well.

The diagnosis hit Morris like an ice bath. At a decidedly unelderly age, his "mid-life" was suddenly very late-life. He was now on a slow but certain trajectory toward forgetting and death. In the turmoil, his on-and-off relationship with a girlfriend fizzled. He was home alone with his books and his dreary thoughts.

At the University of California at Santa Barbara, Morris taught a course called "Human Dignity" and had written his own book on the subject. He crafted a career out of interpreting authors like Viktor Frankl, Martin Buber, and Elie Wiesel. In a superstitious way, Morris hoped that teaching about human suffering might give him a personal bye. "I now see," Morris wrote after his diagnosis, "I thought that teaching this stuff meant, magically, that I'd die by being run over by a truck and never have to face a dramatic challenge to my own human dignity. Oh, well."

His teaching did not shield him from personal tragedy, but it did, evidently, prepare him for it. "For a couple of weeks after the MRI I was struggling with clinical depression. Fortunately, the advice helpful to cancer victims and prisoners-of-war worked for me: Control what you can control, communicate—express your feelings, look death in the face, find meaningful life-tasks and do them, search out and challenge dysfunctional negative thoughts."

Frankl's *Man's Search for Meaning* was central to Morris's work. Before being taken prisoner by the Nazis, Frankl wrote extensively about the human ability to retain dignity under extreme conditions. Then, in the concentration camp, he faced the ultimate personal test of his own ideas. Now, after years of studying him, Morris was echoing Frankl's life. In the freezing, foodless, lice-ridden barracks of Auschwitz, Frankl survived and maintained his dignity. Morris wondered if he could do the same as he was thrown into the dark cave of forgetting.

Just the act of wondering got him off to a good start. What pulled Morris out of his depression was his ability, intellectually, to see how he could retain his essential humanity even as his disease inevitably progressed. "I . . . meditate on an essential core of human connection I can cleave to," he wrote on his Internet home page. "Buddhism identifies three basic interpersonal emotions that even young children enjoy but have great spiritual value. One is compassion. This is the core of human feeling.

"Elie Wiesel wrote, 'You suffer, therefore I am.' It is gratifying to read about the response to distress of the eighteen- to twenty-four-month-old child: 'patting the head, fetching a toy, offering verbal expressions of sympathy, finding an adult to help, and so forth.' When I deteriorate to this level, I too can keep my compassion, and hence my humanity."

Morris did soon regain his emotional balance, and began to forge a new life for himself. He turned back to his books, and to the outside world through his computer, found a new community of people who shared a direct interest in his disease, and bravely opened up a spigot to let his feelings pour out into open view.

"There is pain in forgetfulness," he wrote, "but sometimes there is something delicious in oblivion. Recently I spent some time with the three-year-old grandson of a friend of mine. He has Down's syndrome. I could enjoy sharing with him his friendly little non-verbal world in a way that I never could have before. Not only was my aphasia not a problem—it was like the absence of street noise so I could better savor the music."

Something delicious in oblivion. Could Morris help bridge the widening chasm between the optimistic world of science and the despairing world of sufferers? He knew full well that, as a disease, Alzheimer's is degenerative and incurable. He chose instead to face it as a human condition. In his own forgetting, Morris wanted to find meaning, and hope.

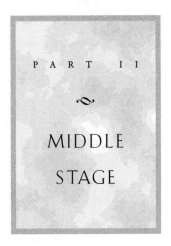

PART II

MIDDLE
STAGE

Chapter 7

FUMBLING FOR

THE NAME OF MY WIFE

◦

On November 12, 1879, two years after he never quite heard, never quite understood, and then entirely forgot Mark Twain's tale of the three famous tramps, Ralph Waldo Emerson, age seventy-six, gave a lecture at the home of Harvard Divinity School professor C. C. Everett. Though Emerson's dementia had steadily progressed over the decade, and he had not written an original lecture in four years, he still occasionally read aloud from old works.

On this particular night, the aging Transcendentalist made a sharply ironic choice of material. Of all things, he read from his twenty-two-year-old essay, "Memory." "Without it," Emerson intoned, "all life and thought were an unrelated succession. As gravity holds matter from flying off into space, so memory gives stability to knowledge; it is the cohesion which keeps things from falling into a lump or flowing in wave. . . .

"Memory performs the impossible for man by the strength of

his divine arms; holds together past and present, beholding both, existing in both, abides in the flowing, and gives continuity and dignity to human life. It holds us to our family, to our friends. Hereby a home is possible; hereby only a new fact has value."

How poignant, and how awful, that as Emerson read aloud these evocative words, his own memory was broken. Much like H.M., he could form no new memories at all. His life from moment to moment *was* an unrelated succession. There was no more continuity except that provided for him by friends and family. At this particular reading, his daughter and caregiver Ellen stood by as a sort of Seeing Eye memory guide. He continually looked up at her to be sure he did not repeat words or sentences.

This was not just an exercise in caution. Without her help, Emerson had recently lost his place many times in lectures, skipped or repeated sentences, and even reread entire pages over again without noticing. In at least one public reading, he had stopped suddenly in the middle of his material and stood silently at the lectern, oblivious. "His words are either not all written or not well remembered," ran a typically disappointed review of these years from the *New Brunswick Daily Times*. ". . . He shows a want of fluency in language, and frequently descends to a tone even fainter than the conversational, and a manner unpleasantly hesitant."

We will never know for sure, of course, whether Emerson was beset with what we now call "Alzheimer's disease." No one bothered to look at the folds of his brain after he died, and if they had they would not have been able to discern anything as detailed as plaques and tangles. Alois Alzheimer was, at the time of Emerson's decline, still a raucous Bavarian youth. Franz Nissl had not yet invented his important tissue stains. Emil Kraepelin had not proposed his radical ideas about autotoxins and organic brain diseases.

We do know from the voluminous record of the details of his life that Emerson had a slow, progressive dementia that in every way appears consistent with the course of typical Alzheimer's disease (albeit on the slower side of the average progression). His illness crept in over time and engendered a slow, almost imperceptible decline. For several years after the trouble first appeared, he was able to hold on to his essential self and treat the memory impairments as disabilities to be worked around, not necessarily any more severe than a broken leg requiring crutches or a wheelchair.

But by the mid-1870s, according to the description of biographer Phillips Russell, Emerson (in his early seventies) had passed into what we now refer to loosely as the middle stages of the disease: "He lived in an internal quietude not to be shattered even by the loudest noises. Outlines and edges were no longer perceptible, and he dwelt in a dreamlike mist which hid from his vision everything that was not intimate and immediately recognizable. . . .

"His love for reading continued, but words ceased to have any intrinsic meaning, and books were sought only for their general tone or flavor. Personality disappeared from all names, and when he sometimes took down from his shelves his own books they possessed a novelty for him exactly like that he would have found in the works of an unknown author. One day when his daughter entered his study, she found him reading very intently in one of his own books. His face revealed his pleasure, and looking up at her, he exclaimed, 'Why, these things are really very good.' "

Because his progression was so slow, Emerson was aware of his deficits for many years. For all of the imperceptible, incremental declines over the months and years in Alzheimer's, one meaningful way to view the disease is as a two-stage disorder: the *awareness* stage and

the *postawareness* stage. Regardless of when (or whether) the actual diagnosis takes place, the sufferer is usually aware for several years that
something is not quite right. He knows that he is forgetting. Then, at
a certain point, usually years into the disease, he no longer knows.

For a long while, Emerson certainly knew. Even before others
perceived any symptoms at all, in fact, he shocked his friends and
family in 1866 (age sixty-three) with a very personal announcement of his imminent decline in the poem "Terminus."

TERMINUS

It is time to be old,
To take in sail:—
The god of bounds,
Who sets to seas a shore,
Come to me in his fatal rounds,
And said: "No more!
No farther shoot
Thy broad ambitious branches, and thy root.
Fancy departs: no more invent,
Contract thy firmament
To compass of a tent.
There's not enough for this and that,
Make thy option which of two;
Economize the failing river,
Not the less revere the Giver,
Leave the many and hold the few.
Timely wise accept the terms,
Soften the fall with wary foot;
A little while

Still plan and smile,
And—fault of novel germs—
Mature the unfallen fruit. . . ."

As the bird trims her to the gale,
I trim myself to the storm of time,
I man the rudder, reef the sail,
Obey the voice at eve obeyed at prime:
"Lowly faithful, banish fear,
Right onward drive unharmed;
The port, well worth the cruise, is near,
And every wave is charmed."

"There he sat," his son Edward later recalled of the chilling moment his father first read the finished poem aloud, "with no apparent abatement of bodily vigor, and young in spirit, recognizing with serene acquiescence his failing forces; I think he smiled as he read. He recognized, as none of us did, that his working days were nearly done."

Sure enough, soon after this formal declaration of decline, expressive aphasia and short-term memory problems surfaced. Groping for the names of famous writers and close friends, for everyday words like "umbrella," and "chair," for new ideas to fill his notebooks and lectures, Emerson gradually settled into a slower, more sheltered life for himself. He cut back on lectures, limited his travel, and worked on a final few projects. "Father has sat quiet in a chair all the forenoon," Ellen wrote to her mother in November 1872, "declaring that idlesse is the business of age, and he loves above all things 'to do noshing' [sic], and that he never before had discovered this privilege of seventy years. . . . also bragging that Edward was a lion over at the

Cathedral yesterday, knew dates and facts like an antiquary, and saying he was glad to have him go to dinners with him, 'so that when I am fumbling for the name of my wife he can remember it for me.'"

Because of who he was and who his friends and colleagues were, Emerson's forgetting was often both personally poignant and historically significant. In a visit by Walt Whitman to Emerson's home in the early 1870s, Emerson turned to Ellen at one point and discreetly asked her, "What is the name of this poet?" Many years later, at the funeral for Henry Wadsworth Longfellow, he is reported to have said of his friend of fifty years, "The gentleman who lies here was a beautiful soul, but I have forgotten his name."

It is a powerful irony that Emerson, of all people, should have lost his memory, not just because he contributed so much to the public discourse on the subjects of intellect, identity, imagination, and the human spirit, but also because he spent his entire life constructing one of the most elaborate external memory systems—in the form of books and journals—of any writer in history. His "Wide World" journals, which he inaugurated in his junior year at Harvard College as "a receptacle of . . . all the luckless raggamuffin Ideas which may be collected & imprisoned hereafter in these pages," ended up filling hundreds of pages and being organized into many distinct subjects and meticulously cross-referenced.

The young Emerson explicitly referred to his brand-new journal as a "tablet to save the wear & tear of weak Memory." It is almost as if Emerson was in conscious preparation throughout his life for the time when he would lose his memory, constructing an elaborate mechanism to fall back on. In his later years, he withdrew to his precious notebooks and more formal writings in order to sustain him as a public figure for the fifteen years that followed the onset of his illness. "I cannot remember anybody's name; not even my recollections of the Latin School," he announced at the centennial celebration of his alma mater. "I have therefore guarded against absolute silence by bringing you a few reminiscences which I have written."

It takes memory, though, to make memory. Once his illness began, his life's work of creating a reservoir of external memory was effectively over. His fertile notebook entries and evocative letters became fewer and terser, accompanied by steady acknowledgments of how his "broken age" had "tied my tongue and hid my memory." His late letters are saturated with basic spelling errors ("som" for some, "claimess" for claims, "tahat" for that), missing words, and repeated words. In sum, he was, by his own third-person declaration, "a man who has lost his wits."

And yet he rarely let on that he was bothered by it. The decision to continue speaking in public perfectly illustrates his exceptional poise. "Things that go wrong at these lectures don't disturb me," Emerson said, "because I know that everyone knows I am worn out and passed by; and that it is only my friends come for friendship's sake to have one last season with me." On another occasion, preparing for a speech, he remarked to Ellen, "A funny occasion it will be—a lecturer who has no idea what he's lecturing about." In light of what Emerson had lost, and *knew* that he had lost, the good humor was remarkable. As Edward had noticed on first hearing "Terminus," the world-famous Emersonian serenity had only intensified, it seemed, with the onset of his dementia.

"Memory" was not an isolated work, but had been conceived and written in his earlier years as a part of what Emerson told his close friend and literary executor James Elliot Cabot was the "chief task" of his life: a series of essays and lectures he called "Natural History of the Intellect." Originally imagined in the 1830s, undertaken in earnest in 1847–48, and reworked in the 1850s, Emerson finally seized the chance to finish the lifelong project as a lecture series for Harvard in the spring of 1870.

Because of their importance, Emerson made sure to invest the necessary time to get them just right. He devised a plan for sixteen lectures, and took most of the winter and spring to organize them. The overall goal was to integrate Transcendentalism with traditional philosophy and science, to bring a spirit of scientific inquiry to the consideration of the nature of mind, of imagination and creativity. "I wish to know the laws of this wonderful power," he wrote, "that I may domesticate it. I observe with curiosity its risings and its settings, illumination and eclipse; its obstructions and its provocations, that I may learn to live with it wisely, court its aid, catch sight of its splendor, feel its approach, hear and save its oracles and obey them."

Alas, he had waited too long. Even with eighteen months of work—he reworked and redelivered the lectures the following spring—he couldn't get it right. After a lifetime of masterly organization, Emerson complained to Thomas Carlyle that he was now finding his work "oppressive." He had lots of good source material, he said, and some good ideas, "but in haste they are misplaced and spoiled." His son Edward observed bluntly that it was "too late for the satisfactory performance of the duty." Emerson wanted desperately to define the parameters of intellect, but his own intellect was no longer up to the task.

After the Harvard ordeal, Emerson was treated to a luxurious seven-week trip westward by John Forbes, the wealthy father of his new son-in-law. A party of twelve piled into a private Pullman train car in Chicago, and were seen off by George Pullman himself. As reported later in a detailed journal by fellow excursioner James Bradley Thayer, Emerson was thrilled to do nothing on this trip but read, relax, talk, eat, and smoke cigars. He developed a happy morning ritual of eating pie before any other foods, and attempted to seduce others into joining him. When, one morning, he was unable to convince anyone within earshot, Emerson playfully slid a knife underneath a slice of pie and, gently tilting it up toward a companion, asked with exaggerated face and voice, "But Mr. ———, what is pie for?"

The first stop was Salt Lake City, where Emerson was introduced to (but was unimpressed by) Mormon leader Brigham Young. Then on to San Francisco, where he admired the sea lions and the California wine. At the San Francisco Unitarian Church, he read aloud his address "Immortality." From there the group traveled to Yosemite. In the Mariposa Grove, Emerson was overwhelmed by the majesty of the giant sequoias, which he called "those gentleman trees."

He was particularly moved by their ability to age with grace, to survive the indignities of fire and other abuse. In thirteen hundred years of life, he remarked, the trees "must have met that danger and every other in turn. Yet they possess great power of resistance."

Continuing their tour of Yosemite, the group came to the majestic Vernal Fall, where someone recited from Longfellow's "Wreck of the Hesperus":

She struck where the white and fleecy waves
Looked soft as carded wool . . .

Emerson was very glad to hear the verse of his friend, but he found it impossible to retain the words in his mind for more than a few moments. "Mr. Emerson gave a pleased nod, and desired it said over again," noted Thayer, evidently oblivious to Emerson's incipient decline. "And then he wished a reference to it when we should get to the hotel. Had he then let Longfellow's poetry pass by him so much?"

In Yosemite, the party on horseback was joined by the young environmentalist John Muir, a great admirer of Emerson. Muir, who would go on to convince Congress to establish Yosemite National Park in 1890, observed that Emerson was as "serene as a sequoia." Emerson was delighted to discover a western protégé. As his group left Yosemite on horseback, Muir recalled: "Emerson lingered in the rear . . . and when he reached the top of the ridge, after all the rest of the party were over and out of sight, he turned his horse, took off his hat and waved me a last good-bye."

*I'm blessed to have a wonderful daughter. . . . I
sent her to school and to college, and now she knows
how to take care of all my business. I depend on her.
I'm in her hands. I'm in my baby phase now, so to
speak. So sometimes I call her my "mumma." Yes,
she's my mumma now.*

—B.
San Diego, California

Chapter 8

BACK TO BIRTH

⌒

Old men are children twice over.

—Aristophanes, 419 B.C.

Queens, New York: Fall 1999

The decline was sure and steady at Freund House, in Queens.

After two years in the group, Doris was now facing more severe aphasia. Her sentences were now so pockmarked with "yeah" in place of other words that it was difficult to tell what she was trying to say much of the time. Even the most productive conversations with Doris involved almost no exchange of information. Over lunch one afternoon, someone mentioned tuna fish. Doris's eyes lit up.

"My mother had a . . . a . . ."

"A recipe?" someone offered.

"Yes . . . she . . . yeah . . . she . . ."

"She had a recipe for tuna fish salad?"

"Yes . . . wonderful."

The thread of conversation ended there. Doris clearly had much more to say on the subject, but translating these thoughts into spoken words was no longer possible. Her world did not collapse entirely on her inability to discuss tuna fish, but to have all potential conversations restricted to a handful of words effectively extinguished her ability to communicate any real thoughts out loud. (One suspected that the intended subject of this un-conversation was not tuna fish, but Doris's mother.)

Rachel, another veteran member of the group, was also deteriorating, and—perhaps blessedly—oblivious to the decline. At the end of one week's session, Irving felt the need to be blunt with her. "Rachel, please talk to your son about getting a review, a medical update. I think it's extremely important."

"On what?"

"On the progression of your dementia."

"Why—do you see something?"

Irving paused briefly to check his frustration. "Yes—I mentioned it to you before that we see a little more progression."

"About remembering? Really?"

"Well, what's happening is that there's even a little bit more of the not-remembering that you're forgetting."

"Not remembering forgetting?"

"Not remembering that *you're* forgetting. In the beginning, you used to come in and say, 'Oh, I forgot.' Now you don't even remember in some of the cases that you forgot."

"Oh."

William was much more confused than before. He got lost on bathroom breaks. Greta had also deteriorated and seemed headed to soon join the middle-stage group for which she had once volunteered.

The group was collapsing. The original vision had been to cycle individual members out of the group as they progressed into the middle stages of the disease—once they were no longer "bothered enough," in Judy's words, to contribute. In practice, this had proven very tough to do, a lot tougher than Irving or Judy had anticipated. Whenever they tried to discuss the exit of one or another member, Irving explained, "The other members jumped on us. They were horrified. 'He's not hurting the group!' they would say."

Even as minds slipped away, the group still held a lot of meaning for these people. They didn't want to let go of their friends, or to acknowledge decline. Shortly before the group disbanded, there was a frank discussion about the future. Or rather, there was an *attempt* by the group leaders at a frank discussion. Stefanie, another group facilitator, tried to prepare the group for what was in store. "This group is a temporary group," she said. "Things may get worse. And you may not remember if they get worse." She raised the possibility of the group retaining the same members, but beginning to meet for a good portion of each day instead of once weekly. This would mark a transition from *self-help* to *day care*.

The group would hear none of it. Even in their impairment, they were sharp enough to know what she was driving at. She was warning them that the early stages were coming to an end.

They weren't ready. The group had been working on coping mechanisms for two years, but simply could not confront the wretched truth head-on. "A lot of people are worse off than me," William protested. "For me, it hasn't changed since I walked in the door. My wife would back me up in that."

"That's right," Greta said, in effect demonstrating her own deteriorating memory and judgment. "He has improved tremendously. He can express himself much better than before." Turning to the issue of her own decline, Greta disputed claims that she had recently been seen walking around Freund House in a state of confusion. "That's just crazy," she insisted. Doris also claimed she wasn't getting any worse.

Denial is an important part of the Alzheimer's experience, very commonly employed as symptoms first appear, or at the time of diagnosis, or at any juncture where a truth is so horrifying that the most emotionally healthy choice is to pretend that it does not exist. The poisonous reality is pushed back into the recesses of the mind and only slowly, in small drips, is it allowed to seep back into consciousness.

It's also customary for denial to fade away and then return again sometime later. This psychological mechanism of last resort can be invoked as often as need be, and in Freund House most of the group members now apparently needed to fall back on it again. For the time being, it didn't matter that they had bravely faced down their disease together for two years. It didn't matter that they had accepted their decreased functioning and voluntarily given up liberties like driving. It didn't matter that they had brought much frustration and despair to the surface. A new awful truth was emerging that was too hard to confront. What they each had glimpsed, if only briefly before suppressing, were the *middle stages*. It wouldn't be so long now before *they* were singing the Barney song and being escorted to the bathroom.

In effect, without anyone quite realizing it, the group had already become a middle-stage group. They no longer knew what had brought them there in the first place, could no longer examine the implications of their own deficits. Of the six of them, Arnie was the only one left still bothered enough to talk about the problems with some candor.

"I think we need to own up to the fact that change occurs," Arnie finally said to his friends in one of their last meetings together. "And in the main, these changes are not positive."

He paused for a moment. "I think I'll leave it at that for now."

Bel Air, California: Fall 1999

Ronald Reagan was also slipping well past the early stages. "Not good" was how Reagan's daughter Maureen characterized his condition in the fifth year following the diagnosis.

The mythic significance of the once "Great Communicator" now steadily unraveling was felt even by Reagan's detractors: Once the most powerful man on earth, he famously confronted the Soviet empire. Now he was caught in a humbling downward spiral, so powerless that he no longer even knew who he was. On the *Today* show, Ann Curry asked Maureen, "Does he remember being President?" She evaded the painful question.

Earlier in the illness, supporters had made much of the fact that Reagan was continuing to go to his office in downtown Los Angeles every day. He played the occasional game of golf and took casual walks in public parks, making himself accessible to passers-by.

Those visits and games were now over, and the Reagans had sold their beloved "Rancho del Cielo" mountaintop retreat. They were hunkering down for some more difficult times. As expected, Reagan's descent had progressed steadily. Friends and family watched his memory lapses become the rule rather than the exception. There was, for example, the day that former Secretary of State George Shultz visited his old boss. In the midst of a casual discussion about politics, Reagan briefly left the room with a nurse. When he returned a few moments later, he took the nurse aside and pointed to Shultz. "Who is that man sitting with Nancy on the couch?" he asked quietly. "I know him. He is a very famous man."

Incidents like these drove him into further isolation. Partly out of simple courtesy to Reagan and partly due to their own personal discomfort, many of his friends stopped visiting when he started having trouble recognizing them.

Then came language stumbles. Over the course of a few years, aphasia crept steadily in and eventually took from him the ability to articulate his thoughts. He could, for a time, still read others' words out loud from a children's storybook. But then that too slipped away.

In visits just after the diagnosis, Maureen and her father would tackle large, three-hundred-piece puzzles. "He and I do jigsaw puzzles together," she said. "He loves doing that. When I was a little girl he used to tell me, 'Do the border first.' Now I sit there and say, 'Dad, do the border first.'"

When the intricate puzzles got too difficult, she brought him simpler puzzles of a hundred pieces or so; then simpler puzzles still, with farm animal scenes. Finally, even those became too challenging. In other homes all over Southern California and elsewhere, tiny children were, day by day, learning to distinguish colors and shapes, gaining in depth perception, improving their hand-eye coordination, slowly gaining confidence as their brains developed to full capacity. Here at 668 St. Cloud Drive, the former President of the United States was heading through that same developmental process in reverse.

The middle stages bring the end of ambiguity. The subtle cues that something was not quite right—so easy to miss a few years ago—

are now bright, self-reflecting signposts of decline, impossible to avoid. Conversation is now pockmarked with lost names and empty recollections. Time and dates have become fungible. Concentration wanes. The mind is now clearly ebbing.

Inside the folds of the brain, the progression is marked by a precise trail of pathology. Now the plaques and tangles have spread well beyond their starting point in the hippocampus. It is not clear how long they germinated there to begin with—*five years? twenty-five years?*—but in a rather short time they have now spread throughout the limbic system and leeched into the temporal, parietal, and frontal lobes of the cerebral cortex. Throughout much of the thinking brain, gooey plaques now crowd neurons from outside the cell membranes, and knotty tangles mangle microtubule transports from inside the cells. All told, tens of millions of synapses dissolve away.

Because the structures and substructures of the brain are so highly specialized, the precise location of the neuronal loss determines what specific abilities will become impaired, and when—like a series of circuit breakers in a large house flipping off one by one:

In the very beginning, when the hippocampus begins to degrade, memory formation fails.

Then, when the nearby amygdala becomes compromised, control over primitive emotions like fear, anger, and craving is disrupted; hostile eruptions and bursts of anxiety may occur all out of proportion to events, or even out of nowhere.

From there, tangles spread outward through much of the rest of the brain, following exactly the same pathways that sensory data travel in a healthy brain. One tangled neuron leads to another tangled neuron leads to another, like a pileup of cars after an accident.

A preponderance of neurons in the brain, 80 percent, are devoted to so-called higher-order processing—finely tuned perception, analysis, comparison, recollection, anticipation, and abstraction—with the small remainder left for perceiving stimuli and behavioral response. Of the higher-order association areas, the temporal lobes, just inside from the ear on either side of the brain, are the closest to the hippocampus and therefore the next to bear the brunt of Alzheimer's. Temporal lobes are responsible for primary organization of sensory input, for processing language, and for ecstatic feelings of spiritual transcendence. A healthy temporal lobe stimulated by an electrical probe can spontaneously produce powerful religious images, along with specific memories of songs and vivid hallucinations of friends' faces. Not surprisingly, auditory and visual hallucinations are not uncommon in the middle and later stages of Alzheimer's.

Next in line are the parietal and frontal lobes. The parietal lobes, on top of the brain, extending to the rear, handle touch, vibration, pain, and spatial awareness. They enable the control of limbs and eyes, and the recognition of objects by physical contact. Damage to the sensory portions of the parietal lobe can cause *agnosia,* the inability to understand the source or meaning of touch. The patient becomes an island, floating apart from the external world.

When tangles finally reach the frontal lobes, which help to manage the retrieval of already formed memories, identity itself begins to vanish. A lifetime of memories exists in constellations all throughout the brain, but without a reliable system of retrieval, they'll sit dormant forever. (The temporal lobe also plays a crucial role in accessing semantic—intellectual—memories.)

The frontal lobes are also where most of what we consider intelligent thought takes place. Here is where massive amounts of sensory data are brought together, integrated and analyzed, where the brain makes sense of unfolding events, contrasts them with previous experience, adapts future plans based on that contrast. Once the frontal lobes come under heavy fire, the will itself begins to unravel, and, as one Alzheimer's text puts it, "the chain of mental contents is no longer guided by a logically valid executive program." The sufferer and her family cannot continue to treat her forgetfulness as a liability that can be overcome with Post-it Notes. It now becomes the dominant force in the patient's life, a major disability.

The list of cognitive abilities that dwindle in the middle stages of the disease is difficult for a cognitively healthy person to fully comprehend, because the functions lost are so basic. Memories are erased not just of specific events (grocery shopping last night), but general concepts learned long ago (what groceries *are*). Other central competencies that wither include:

The ability to understand simple questions, instructions, gestures

The ability to follow a conversation, or even to keep track of one's own words or thoughts

The ability to place oneself in the right time of day, or the right time of year

The ability, even the desire, to plan for the future

The ability to choose one's own clothes and draw one's own bath

The ability to recognize one's friends and relatives, or even one's spouse

The capacity for awareness (In these years, the sufferer loses all awareness of his or her condition. Introspection vanishes. This is known as *anosognosia*.)

Perhaps the only practical way to understand such a cata-strophic loss is to imagine oneself as a very young child who has not yet developed these abilities in the first place. "All actions of the bodie and minde are weakened and growne feeble," a physician of King Henry IV of France said of old age in 1599. "The senses are dull, the memorie lost, and the judgment failing so that they become as they were in the infancie." That same century, Erasmus suggested even more fully:

Old men are more eagerly delighted with children, and they, again, with old men. . . . For what difference between them, but that the one has more wrinkles and years upon his head than the other? Otherwise, the brightness of their hair, toothless mouth, weakness of body, love of mild, broken speech, chatting, toying, forgetfulness, inadvertency, and briefly, all other their actions agree in everything. And by how much the nearer they approach to this old age, by so much they grow backward into the likeness of children, until like them they pass from life to death, without any weariness of the one, or sense of the other.

Five hundred years later, caregivers use the same comparisons. "Not long after my [recently diagnosed] mother came to live with us, our daughter also came with her fourteen-month-old son," Daisy from Raceland, Kentucky, told fellow caregivers via the Alzheimer List. "I find that what works with him also works with Mom, and they give the same angelic smile when pleased. On the downside, there is also the same tantrum at times and stamp of the foot. What I do to safety-proof the house for the baby also works as Nana-proofing, for the most part. The same behavior-address-ing works as well. Often when he is cranky, it is due to some other influence—just like her. I have learned to read between the lines at both ends of the age spectrum. Sadly enough, he is learning to potty train at the time when my mom is losing that ability."

In 1980, New York University neurologist Barry Reisberg realized that the Alzheimer's-childhood analogy is not just anecdotal—that it could be measured scientifically. Reisberg was a pioneer in defining stages and substages of Alzheimer's, trying to gain a much more precise understanding of the disease's trajectory. The more he drilled down on the exact order of abilities lost, the more he was impressed by the comparison to child development. He began to notice that there were precise inverse relationships between stages of Alzheimer's disease and phases of child development in the areas of cognition, coordination, language, feeding, and behavior.

He documented these observations in comparison charts. Placed side by side, the sequences of abilities gained and lost nearly perfectly mirror one another.

CHILD DEVELOPMENT

Age	Acquired Ability
1–3 months	Can hold up head
2–4 months	Can smile
6–10 months	Can sit up without assistance
1 year	Can walk without assistance
1 year	Can speak one word
15 months	Can speak 5–6 words
2–3 years	Can control bowels
3–4.5 years	Can control urine
4 years	Can use toilet without assistance
4–5 years	Can adjust bath water temperature
4–5 years	Can put on clothes without assistance

5–7 years	Can select proper clothing for occasion or season
8–12 years	Can handle simple finances
12+ years	Can hold a job, prepare meals, etc.

ALZHEIMER'S DISEASE

Stage	Lost Ability
1	No difficulty at all
2	Some memory trouble begins to affect job/home
3	Much difficulty maintaining job performance
4	Can no longer hold a job, prepare meals, handle personal finances, etc.
5	Can no longer select proper clothing for occasion or season
6a	Can no longer put on clothes properly
6b	Can no longer adjust bath water temperature
6c	Can no longer use toilet without assistance
6d	Urinary incontinence
6e	Fecal incontinence
7a	Speech now limited to six or so words per day
7b	Speech now limited to one word per day
7c	Can no longer walk without assistance
7d	Can no longer sit up without assistance
7e	Can no longer smile
7f	Can no longer hold up head

In neurological exams, there were similarly precise inverse relationships in EEG activity, brain glucose metabolism, and neurologic reflexes. The only possible conclusion Reisberg could draw was that, like the winding and unwinding of a giant ball of string, Alzheimer's unravels the brain almost exactly in the reverse order as it develops from birth. Clearly, the phenomenon warranted more formal study, and a name. Reisberg called it "retrogenesis"—*back to birth.*

Retrogenesis is not a perfect reversal, of course—not literally the unwiring of the brain, neuron by neuron, according to some bizarre genetic instruction booklet. But the deconstruction is remarkably similar to the construction. What researchers realized in delving further into this comparison was that Alzheimer's degeneration followed the opposite pattern of brain *myelinization*—the insulation of nerve axons with a white myelin sheath in order to boost the strength of their signals.

Imagine a house thoroughly wired for electricity and phone use, but without any wire insulation—all the unprotected copper wires wrapped up together and touching one another. Infants are born with billions of neurons but almost no myelin insulation protecting these neurons, rendering them virtually useless. As neurons in various regions of the brain become insulated during child development, generating the famous "white matter" of the brain, these regions are *brought online,* made effective.

We know much about child brain development, thanks to J. L. Conel, a Boston neuropathologist who in 1939 began painstakingly dissecting the brains of deceased children. Over nearly thirty years, he examined the cerebral cortex from brains aged one month, three months, six months, fifteen months, two years, four years, and six years.

What he discovered comported with every parent's experience of their growing child: The first neurons to gain myelin insulation are in the primary motor area, enabling gross movements of the hands, arms, upper trunk, and legs. Next come the primary sensory area neurons in the parietal lobe, bringing gross touch sensations online. After that comes some development of the occipital lobe for visual acuity, followed by the temporal lobe for auditory processing. Gradually, the association areas are then formed, allowing the brain to make more and more sense of the perceptions being registered. Symbolic processing areas then begin to develop slowly, enabling language. Eventually the frontal cortex matures, enabling concentration, abstract thought, and the ability to plan.

One of the very last structures in the brain to be covered in protective myelin is the hippocampus, making it one of the last places to work effectively. This is why children generally don't have any permanent memories prior to age three (although the amygdala can store some very early emotional memories).

The reverse myelinization process of Alzheimer's begins with the most recent and least-myelinated brain region—the hippocampus. From there it moves to the next least-myelinated, and so on. In this one respect, at least, the disease process makes sense. It has its own logic.

For better or worse, the strange notion of reverse childhood turns out to be the best map we have to understand the terrain of Alzheimer's. Think of a teenager you know today and try to imagine her rapid development suddenly halting and beginning to reverse course at roughly the same developmental pace. Over the next twelve years or so, she loses everything she has gained, slowly and steadily.

First, she begins to lose her sense of humor and fashion sense. Now, watch her ambitions become less and less pronounced; then begin to peel away what she has learned from school and parents and peers and television over the last couple of years. Her sense of the world and her place in it fades away. Week by week she becomes not more but less articulate, less independent. She loses her Dairy Queen job because she has forgotten what "ice cream" and "cone" mean, and cannot add very well. As time ticks forward but seems to be going backward, she is now having a hard time picking out her own clothes; most of what she is saying you can no longer understand, and vice versa.

Further imagine your backwards teenager traversing her way back to infancy, to her very first day of birth, her first breath, and you have a surprisingly good grasp of the unraveling of mind, soul, and body that Alzheimer's inflicts on a person. Every skill, feeling, and fact that the patient has learned slowly, satisfyingly, is being steadily erased as if by some sort of cosmic punishment.

The child analogy understandably rankles many caregivers. They are deeply offended at the suggestion that their mother or father or husband or wife is now to be regarded as a mere child. It feels like the ultimate insult one could inflict on someone. Not yet fully formed, children are regarded as incomplete persons. We love them, of course, and recognize them as human beings, but we do not fully trust them. We assume a certain responsibility and even moral superiority over them. To assume this same posture toward a parent or grandparent who has stood for a lifetime in a position of moral authority is a sad and sour thing. It is tragic and demoralizing to suddenly strip our esteemed elders of their authority and reposition them as untrustworthy and intellectually inferior.

But the comparison is a valid, and even necessary, one to make. Here is an instance where scientists fighting disease and caregivers trying to make peace with a human tragedy can come to some common ground: the science of retrogenesis can help caregivers forge a new understanding and appreciation of what their loved ones are going through. Caregivers like Daisy from Raceland find the prism of second childhood helps ease both their chores and psychological strain. By viewing their loved ones as reverting back to childhood abilities and mentalities, caregivers can establish a more humane formula for their care. Whether or not it feels demeaning, retrogenesis can be *instructive*.

As reverse childhood came to seem more and more medically relevant, Alzheimer's researchers in the 1990s began dredging up everything known about developmental biology and psychology to test it for the possible application to their field. Colleagues of Reisberg, for instance, decided to test on severely demented patients a specially modified version of the Ordinal Scales of Psychological Development (OSPD), a test originally designed for infants and toddlers and based on Jean Piaget's theories of development.

This kind of ultra-basic testing had never been done before on Alzheimer's victims. The testers stripped down the OSPD so that it required no vocal abilities at all. They designed it to measure five rudimentary skills:

1. *Visual pursuit and object permanence.* Can the patient keep track of an object moving through an arc of 180 degrees?

2. *Means-ends.* Can the patient reach out for an object, causing an event to occur?

3. *Causality.* Does the patient react to a spectacle with an expression of understanding, such as a smile or frown?

4. *Spatial relations.* Can the patient adjust her vision between two objects?

5. *Schemes.* Can the patient visually inspect an object in her hands?

The experiment worked beautifully. Using criteria initially crafted to measure infant development, the researchers found what they called "residual cognitive capacities" in advanced-stage Alzheimer's patients who had previously been considered untestable.

The implications of this discovery are enormous for the development of caregiving strategies for middle and late-stage Alzheimer's patients. With new layers of understanding what patients are capable of and what they are no longer capable of at any specific stage of the disease, caregivers can be much more *prepared.* They can train themselves, in effect, to be competent reverse parents—not a skill that comes naturally.

If an Alzheimer's sufferer, for example, has progressed to the point where he is trying to put on an undershirt over a sweater, it now could be easily discerned that he has slipped into stage 6a of Alzheimer's, which, via retrogenesis, can be reasonably correlated to age four. Knowing that, one can also infer that the patient has now slid into what Piaget called the "Preoperational" stage. He is still able to represent reality through symbols (to count on his fingers, for example), but he is no longer able to rely on a solid foundation of logic (to understand the importance of going to bed early if he has to get up early the next day). He is also on the cusp of losing the sense that his point of view is distinct from that of others.

Properly utilized, the lens of retrogenesis can allow caregivers to enter the world of Alzheimer's disease with a broad new understanding. Caregivers can hone a sense that something coherent is happening, rather than what looks to the uninitiated like a random and unintelligible breakdown. Anyone who understands child-hood can grasp the basic concept of reverting to that state, of developing in reverse. It helps make Alzheimer's caregiving a more human endeavor.

In *Max's New Suit,* Rosemary Wells's popular children's book, Max the young rabbit bumbles through the task of dressing himself. His older sister Ruby tries to teach him, but Max still puts his pants on over his head and his shirt on his legs. It is written about, and for, a very young child, but will work just as well in any nursing home (where between 60 and 80 percent of the patients are suffering from dementia). The world of children's literature turns out to be highly relevant to Alzheimer's. In Barbara M. Joosse's book, *Mama, Do You Love Me?,* to give another example, a little girl asks, "What if I ran away?"

"Then I would be worried," her mother answers.

"What if I stayed away and sang with the wolves and slept in a cave?"

"Then, Dear One, I would be very sad. But still, I would love you."

". . . What if I turned into a polar bear, and I was the meanest bear you ever saw and I had sharp, shiny teeth, and I chased you into your tent and you cried?"

"Then I would be very surprised and very scared. But still, inside the bear, you would be you, and I would love you."

The book is about a child exploring the boundaries of unconditional love. But in a home tainted by Alzheimer's disease, it also comes off as a perfect parable for the anxieties of both sufferer and caregiver. The sufferer wants to know, *What will happen when I become a real burden?* The caregiver wonders how bad the wandering, stubbornness, irritability, and bursts of snarling anger will become. As the illness progresses, she will struggle to look through the *disease* and recognize the *person* inside.

Not surprisingly, caregivers report that Alzheimer's patients in the middle and later stages find a tremendous comfort in children's books and music. They also like stuffed animals and dolls. The child's world—nurturing, safe, colorful, full of soft edges and sweet treats—is what middle-stage patients crave. "Mom enjoys car rides," says Pam from Baton Rouge, Louisiana. "It doesn't matter where we go or if we go anywhere other than drive around. She likes to look at the trees and anything green. . . . She got to the point where being in the store didn't work out too well. Now we still go but not to accomplish anything. We walk the mall and window-shop. If we go in a store it's like the Disney Store or a toy store to look at the stuffed animals. We look at the plants and decorations. We get ice cream."

The daughter has become the mother, the mother the daughter. Catastrophic disease often alters roles, but only Alzheimer's disease can fully reverse them.

Some days are so normal, I am guilty of thinking, "Well maybe he really isn't . . . ?" Then, to bring me back to reality, he wraps all my Tupperware in masking tape. Today, he went out to his workshop to "fix" an old LP record player, got side-tracked and ended up in the yard with a pair of clippers where he decimated my carefully cultivated rosemary bushes.

He was so proud of what he had done. Got rid of those weeds! Oh, well, the air was redolent with the aroma of rosemary. Rosemary is supposed to be the herb for remembrance. Maybe I should rub it in his hair.

—M.V.
Ft. Pierce, Florida

Chapter 9

NATIONAL INSTITUTE OF ALZHEIMER'S

❧

In the 1960s, public officials began to notice something: There were more old people than ever, and they voted. The portion of the population living to eighty-five or beyond had tripled since 1900, and the elderly were becoming conspicuous for the first time in human history. A new lobbying organization, the American Association of Retired Persons (AARP), founded in 1958, was on its way to making senior citizens the most powerful interest group in American politics. In 1965, the U.S. government established Medicare, a sweeping federal program designed to protect every citizen "against the ravages of illness in his old age."

Around the same time, researchers were finally uncovering the true significance of one of those illnesses. At the Albert Einstein College of Medicine in New York, neuropathologists Robert Terry and Robert Katzman were shocked to see plaques and tangles turning up in so many brain samples. "We found Alzheimer's cases coming out of the woodwork," said Terry. "It was very common, and that surprised us. We didn't know that Alzheimer's was so common. Everybody thought that senile dementia was due to small artery disease."

After Katzman's sixty-four-year-old mother-in-law was diagnosed with Alzheimer's, he finally realized the larger hidden problem—the very problem that Meta Neumann had tried to expose two decades earlier. "It became obvious to me that Alzheimer's disease was a single entity regardless of age of onset," he said. "When I did simple multiplication, it became evident that this was a very important public health problem."

According to Katzman's calculations, Alzheimer's was already one of the leading causes of death in the United States, probably already killing 100,000 people per year in the U.S. alone. Those numbers would only get larger as the population aged even more.

The world had ignored Meta Neumann in 1953, but now people were ready to listen. Katzman's speeches and editorials in the early 1970s struck a chord with the medical community, which finally seemed open to the idea of senile dementia being a *disease*. As society aged, mores were shifting. So many people were living so long that senility didn't feel so normal or acceptable anymore. A critical mass of doctors began to *prefer* to see senility as a disease. The medical establishment was now ready to take on the moral challenge of Alzheimer's, to make a commitment to intervention.

But how? Researchers didn't know much more about Alzheimer's in the 1960s than they had in 1910. Robert Terry used an electron microscope to observe plaques and tangles at magnifications of up to one hundred times greater than Alois Alzheimer's original view, enabling him to begin to map out a cellular "ultrastructure" of the disease. But his extreme close-ups still did not reveal a cause, or even indicate whether plaques or tangles were closer to the root of the problem. Further progress would require a major new investment in the science of aging and the biology of Alzheimer's. In the early 1970s, health experts called on Congress to establish a National Institute on Aging.

The National Institute of Health (NIH) was established by Congress in 1930, but it wasn't until the late 1940s that two Washington activists began to transform it into the world's foremost center for medical research. Florence Mahoney was a former newspaper reporter and the wealthy widow of the publisher of the *Miami Herald;* Mary Lasker was cofounder of the prestigious Albert Lasker Medical Research Awards, the recipients of which commonly go on to win the Nobel Prize. Together, the two women devised a lobbying technique known as "the politics of anguish," coaxing friends in government and the media into focusing on the ravages of particular diseases rather than general scientific research.

This disease-by-disease approach converted dispassionate intellectual curiosity into a series of personal crusades. Politicians effortlessly gravitated to a war on cancer. They found it easy to convince their constituents that everyone's grandchildren should be spared from polio. Between 1950 and 1960, thanks to Mahoney and Lasker, the NIH budget grew from $46.3 million to $400 million—and became the National Institutes of Health.

Questions about aging research, though, caused a rift in the activist duo. In the early 1970s, Mahoney became convinced that the NIH needed a distinct institute to focus exclusively on the problems of the fastest growing part of the population. Lasker disagreed. She felt that the best way to deal with the problems of aging was to continue the fight against heart disease and cancer. Mahoney went ahead on her own, helping to push the Research on Aging Act of 1972 through Congress. It was vetoed that year by Richard Nixon.

Congress did not have the votes to override Nixon's veto, but two years later it unexpectedly had a different sort of leverage. In 1973, the Nixon White House began to fall under the siege of the Watergate investigation. By 1974, impeachment seemed a very real possibility, giving Congress the upper hand on Nixon. When the Research on Aging Act of 1972 was passed essentially unchanged by Congress as the Research on Aging Act of 1974, Nixon—desperate not to provoke the representatives controlling his fate—signed it. It became law on May 31, 1974, less than two months before he left office.

Robert Butler, the first director of the new National Institute on Aging (NIA), immediately signaled that he intended to make Alzheimer's a top priority. He hired the neurobiologist Zaven Khachaturian to wage war on Alzheimer's.

Khachaturian had been interested in the biology of memory since his days as an undergraduate at Yale in the late 1950s. Later, at the University of Pittsburgh's psychiatric department, he had started to focus on the physiology of forgetting and dementia. Along the way, he also felt the personal sting of the disease: His mother suffered from a progressive memory loss that he later came to suspect was Alzheimer's. "She was increasingly unable to remember the names of people she had just met," he recalled. "She repeated the same questions again and again, as though they had just popped into her head for the first time." Her forgetting progressed slowly; for many years before she died (from heart disease), she was lucid enough to question her son about his memory research—and yet unable to remember much of what he said.

As his mother drifted away, Khachaturian fashioned himself as the brigadier general of the modern war on Alzheimer's. Over two decades, he recruited top researchers, designed research paradigms, collaborated on funding proposals and translated the science to Congress and the public. "I started a crystal growing in all of the major areas—a group on neurochemistry, a group on protein chemistry, one on the infection hypothesis, and one on genetics. I tried to get all the major ideas started because I had no idea which one was going to pay off.

"I also purposefully tried to recruit people who had opposing points of view. There were royal battles. But since I was doling out the money on behalf of the government, my attitude was that I was going to get all these folks started on a level playing field."

The organic crystal quickly grew into a research palace. In the first five years, NIA research funding rose from $19.3 million to $70 million. By 1985, the NIA had established ten federally funded Alzheimer's disease research centers—a brainchild of Khachaturian—to coordinate clinical, behavioral, and laboratory research. The battle was on.

The public also started to learn about Alzheimer's for the first time in the late 1970s, from doctors and the media. Rita Hayworth was diagnosed in 1980. That same year, the syndicated columnist Abigail Van Buren printed an aching letter about Alzheimer's in her "Dear Abby" column. In 1982, President Reagan conferred the first of his two giant spotlights on the disease by proclaiming November "National Alzheimer's Month."

George Glenner, chief of molecular pathology at NIH and one of Zaven Khachaturian's star recruits to Alzheimer's research, was invited to the White House for the proclamation. As one of the few Alzheimer's experts present, Glenner was given the task of explaining the little-known disease to Reagan.

"The President looked at me and asked, 'What is Alzheimer's disease?' " Glenner recalled. "I explained that it was tangles and plaques that form in gray matter that keep neuronal cells from being nourished. Well, he looked at me and smiled.

" 'All I know is that my mother died in a nursing home and she didn't recognize me at the end,' he said."

Turning Alzheimer's into a household word was an official part of the political research strategy—using the "politics of anguish" as a tool to raise as much public interest and as many public dollars as possible. But there was a fallout from educating masses of people about a haunting and incurable disease. While scientists regarded Alzheimer's as a great new frontier, an exciting challenge, the public was left merely bewildered and anxious.

The new message was oppressive and hopeless: Old people did not sometimes gently "go senile." Rather, they were afflicted with a disease. No one was immune from this disease. The cause was unknown. There was no foreseeable treatment or cure.

The longer one lived, the greater one's chance would be of getting this disease.

Inadvertently, health officials had created two new problems: a new disease and a new cultural demon. The public needed more. To exist alongside the frightening unknown is often simply intolerable. In order to cope, we all need some comprehensible grasp of events outside our control, whether or not the interim explanations turn out to be true.

Senility had been plenty frightening to people before it was called Alzheimer's disease, of course, and people had always sought comforting explanations for it. One ancient Roman superstition held that old people lost their memories as a result of reading epitaphs on tombstones. A tenth-century Arabic medical text blamed senility on cold, tenacious phlegm in the brain. Then, in the seventeenth century, the suspicion shifted to an excess of internal humidity—followed by a counter-theory that the real culprit was excessive dryness.

In 1984, amidst the surge in popular interest, the Nobel laureate Torsten Wiesel offered an irresistible, if accidental, explanation for senile dementia at a New York City cocktail party. In casual conversation, Wiesel made a vague reference to a possible link between aluminum and Alzheimer's disease.

Immediately, ears around Wiesel perked up. *What's this? A plain explanation for Alzheimer's disease?* The remark spread like a virus, and mutated. Word got out, incorrectly, that Wiesel was about to publish a paper proving that aluminum causes Alzheimer's disease.

Even (perhaps especially) in our modern age dominated by science and reason, people need to fill the void of ignorance with something; Wiesel's suggestion clicked, for many, with their intuitive suspicion of modern life. *Of course* we are killing ourselves with the invisible residue of progress—radioactivity, pollution, trace molecules from the plastics and metals that define the contours of our daily existence. *Alzheimer's from aluminum:* a new disease for an advanced civilization. People may not have understood the link exactly, but somehow it made perfect sense. A powerful myth was born.

Suddenly, in New York and spreading elsewhere, people began to toss out their aluminum cookware, their aluminum-laden antiperspirants, and their aluminum-based antacids. The Aluminum Association went on the defensive, insisting to reporters that its foils and saucepans were safe. But the image of aluminum-as-brain-toxin stuck. The link between aluminum and dementia became the one "fact" about Alzheimer's disease that every literate adult seemed to know.

The truth was less captivating than the buzz. Aluminum wasn't a cause of Alzheimer's disease, but an effect. High concentrations of aluminum had indeed been found in victims' brains during autopsy; this meant, though, that something had gone wrong with the filter system, called the "blood-brain barrier," that was supposed to keep such elements out of the brain. Everyone ingests significant amounts of aluminum and other metals from the water, air, and many natural foods. In healthy individuals, these complex elements are safely kept out of the brain, where they would do serious damage.

Researchers couldn't figure out why the blood-brain barrier was being compromised, but it was clear enough that avoiding aluminum pots in order to escape Alzheimer's disease was like refusing to drink out of glass containers because someone might come along and break one over your head: The hazard has nothing whatever to do with ordinary use.

It turned out that Wiesel was not even working on Alzheimer's disease, let alone writing a paper on the dangers of aluminum. When reached for comment by a *Washington Post* reporter, he quickly corrected the misimpression and laughed nervously about the unintentional power of his offhand remark, vowing to be more careful.

What of the people, though, who would not make such a vow?

> INTERVIEWER: So you're saying [Alzheimer's] is not just a brain problem?
>
> DR. RICHARD SCHULZE: Oh, no, not at all. [One patient of mine] came out of it by cleansing his bowel. . . . Some people are there because they are toxically poisoned from the outside. Some people are toxically poisoned from the [inside]. Or it's from emotional strain they couldn't deal with. Some from metal poisonings like aluminum. I've met people who were just overdosed with aluminum from the fluorides to the antacids to aluminum pots and pans. So I think you have to take each case individually. . . . There's no such thing as Alzheimer's disease, that's what I've discovered. Every person has a different story, from mothballs to aluminum, to "I couldn't handle my life because my husband was cheating on me."
>
> —from *The Last Chance Health Report*, edited by Sam Biser

A popular figure in the world of alternative healing, Dr. Schulze is not a medical doctor. Among other credentials, he has a doctorate in herbology from the School of Natural Healing, an unaccredited correspondence school based in Orem, Utah. He sells books, audiotapes, videotapes, and several "original" herbal formulas to combat a wide variety of diseases. He offers a special tea for dementia patients:

15 parts ginkgo leaf

1 part gotu kola herb

1 part galamus root

1 part rosemary flowers

1 part kola nut

1 part cayenne pepper, the hottest you can get

One teaspoon of herbs to a cup of tea. Six cups per day.

Schulze is not alone, of course, in supplying the wishful world with simple explanations and cures for Alzheimer's. Others have blamed fluoride in the drinking water, amalgam tooth fillings, pasteurized milk, green tea, refined flour, polished rice, gallstones, and tiny parasites in the colon. Among the alleged cures: unrefined sea salt, flaxseed oil, lemonade (in the morning), miso, mistletoe, red grapes, turmeric, essiac tea, chlorela algae, barley grass, shark cartilage, olive leaf extract, acupuncture, electromagnetic pulse therapy, hyperbaric oxygen therapy, ultraviolet blood irradiation, and—another Richard Schulze suggestion—deep, painful massage of the feet.

A 1995 survey indicated that more than half of Alzheimer's sufferers have tried at least one of these therapies. Twenty percent have tried three or more of them. The impulse is certainly understandable. A relentless, degenerative disease eats away at a person's cognition while most well-meaning doctors throw up their hands and declare that there is virtually nothing to be done. Legitimate suspicions arise: These doctors are Western—what about thousands of years of Eastern wisdom? What about substances that the famously slow U.S. Food and Drug Administration hasn't yet approved? On the Internet, there is excited talk about drugs available only in Europe or Asia. With seemingly little to lose, sufferers and caregivers may grasp for anything that glitters.

Buyers should beware, though. Conventional science, indeed, does not have all the answers; any serious Alzheimer's researcher would be the first to acknowledge that. But how do the explanations of others hold up under scrutiny?

Few of Schulze's claims are upheld by medically supported fact. Alzheimer's *is* a recognizable disease, with a predictable set of symptoms and recognizable pathology. No single case of Alzheimer's disease has ever been cured by a bowel cleansing, or psychotherapy, or any other treatment. The cause of Alzheimer's is not yet known, but there is considerable evidence that it is caused by a combination of genetic and environmental factors.

Schulze's specific list of environmental culprits—though terrifying to the layman—is not confirmed by any serious scholarship. Reputable studies of fluoride, amalgam tooth fillings, aluminum, and other popularly suspected substances have so far come up empty.

In the end, though, Schulze's supreme confidence is the best clue to his illegitimacy; genuine scientists speak in more tentative terms, always careful not to overstep the bounds of what has been proven. Much is known about Alzheimer's, but the many unanswered questions and its incurability demand humility, not the pretension of certainty.

As for Schulze's tea: While heavy doses of gingko have been shown to have some very mild effects in ameliorating some of the symptoms of dementia, the effects always appear to be temporary and do not appear to slow its progress. The final ingredient in Schulze's dementia tea, moreover, should raise eyebrows. No reputable medical studies show that cayenne powder has a demonstrable effect on the brain, and the quantity he is prescribing will make any beverage fiery hot. Imagine the effect of slipping a copious amount of red-hot pepper into the drink of an unsuspecting patient who is only half-lucid and has no powers of communication left. Now imagine doing that six times a day.

A year after George Glenner helped explain Alzheimer's to Ronald Reagan at the White House, he delivered the first major combat victory in Zaven Khachaturian's war on Alzheimer's. In 1983, he unlocked the molecular structure of *beta-amyloid,* the main component of plaques.

Laboratory science had improved considerably since the day of Alois Alzheimer. In 1906, the forefront of brain research was the ability to view cells and their components at a magnification of several hundred times. Alzheimer could see the outlines of the plaques and tangles; he could draw them, count them, describe them, stand in awe of them. But he could not learn much about them. He could not get inside of them and see what they were made of, or understand how they were altering the surrounding tissue.

By the time Glenner came to the subject, the view of plaques and tangles through a light microscope was akin to looking at New York City from the Goodyear blimp: a vivid scene, intriguing, but not very enlightening. What interested modern researchers was the street-level view, and the scene behind closed doors—the nearly hidden molecular and chemical processes cooking inside. From the blimp, plaques were large, dense, menacing-looking clouds of foreign matter. Up close, Glenner could see that tiny strips of *beta-amyloid,* a sticky, insoluble protein fragment, were sticking to one another like wisps of used packing tape torn from a package as it was opened in haste. The tape strips spilled onto the floor, stuck to dust, to hair, to each other. After a while, they started to gum up the whole room.

Glenner decoded the molecular composition of the starchlike beta-amyloid (from *amylum,* the Latin word for starch), which in turn enabled other researchers to find its source. This was the foot in the door that many other researchers had been waiting for. "George came along and sequenced the protein," recalled Zaven Khachaturian, "and, oh my God, it was like the floodgates opened." The story of how plaques become plaques was finally unraveled.

Plaques were caused by a chemical accident, the defective breakdown of a benign substance called amyloid precursor protein (APP) that lives throughout the body—in the brain, heart, kidneys, lungs, spleen, and intestines—and has some still-unknown role in cellular function. As a part of routine function, APP regularly gets broken down into much smaller soluble components and washed away with other decomposed tissue and chemicals. But under some mysterious conditions, the breaking-apart doesn't work right, and out come sticky shards of beta-amyloid. As they stick to each other and attract other detritus—fragments of dead and dying neurons—they slowly form into dense, misshapen clumps: plaques.

Three years later, in 1986, the tangles were also decoded. Researchers discovered that they were made up of another contaminated protein called *tau,* which normally serves as railroad ties for a tracklike structure that transports nutrients and other important molecules throughout the cell body of every neuron. The tangled tau had somehow become hyperphosphorylated—corrupted by several extra molecules of phosphorus. Without the railroad ties, the tracks had no integrity. They got bent into a twisted mess.

Imagine some metal-chewing gremlin working its way down railroad tracks, chewing up the steel ties (the tau). Then, under the weight of the train (the nutrients being transported), the tracks buckle. The damage is compounded as the train continues to speed along, causing a mass of twisted wreckage all along the tracks.

Inside the neuron, the twisted debris gets worse and worse, as the filaments keep twisting around one another. Communication and cell nourishment are at first compromised, and then drop off to nothing; the neuron cannot sustain itself in any way and begins to wither. The cell membranes collapse, and every part of the neuron—the long axon that is responsible for sending out signals to other neurons, the short, branchlike dendrites responsible for receiving signals from other neurons, and everything else—disintegrates. The thousands of synapses, each representing a fragment of a memory, vanish like a plane flying over the Bermuda Triangle. At the end, there is no trace that the neuron itself ever existed—except for one thing. All that's left, if a pathologist stains the tissue just right, is a small clump of what neuropathologists call "ghost tangles." There, a neuron once stood.

A decade after Zaven Khachaturian had gone hunting for new Alzheimer's researchers, here were the first big payoffs. It was suddenly a very exciting time to be in the field. The modern race to understand Alzheimer's and defeat it had begun in earnest. But many more hazards lay ahead.

George Glenner fell mysteriously ill about ten years after his important breakthrough with beta-amyloid. He had shortness of breath and fatigue, and when doctors started doing tests, none of the obvious possibilities checked out.

When they finally discovered what it was, the entire Alzheimer's research community took a shudder: Glenner had somehow contracted a very rare disease called systemic senile amyloid-osis—the unexplained proliferation of amyloid proteins through-out the body, clogging up his heart and other organs. It was, in a sense, Alzheimer's disease of the body.

"How I got this? We don't know," Glenner serenely said to a reporter shortly before he died. "It's just one of those mysteries." Whatever the ultimate explanation, it looked like more than a co-incidence. It certainly seemed that he was inadvertently sacrificing his own body for the sake of scientific discovery.

Just before he died in 1995, Glenner was asked if he thought there would be a cure for Alzheimer's.

"Of course," he said.

I have really struggled with the honesty issue. What do you say to someone who sits on her bed and says that she has never stayed out overnight without letting her parents know where she is? What do you say to someone who thinks she is a teacher and if she doesn't get home and into her classroom there will be a whole class of children left unattended? What do you say to someone who thinks she has no money to pay bills and will lose everything she owns if she doesn't get home to a job that you know she has been retired from for years? I couldn't find any reason for telling her over and over that she has a horrible terrible degenerating disease that was making her feel the way she does.

I found that she became less anxious if I just listened to what she was saying and feeling. Sometimes saying nothing was better than anything I could say. Telling her that I would take care of some of these things put her a bit more at ease. It may feel better for me to verbalize the facts, but what she needs is comfort and security—not the truth. The truth won't change anything.

—N.B.
Merrimack, New Hampshire

Chapter 10

TEN THOUSAND FEET,
AT TEN O'CLOCK AT NIGHT

❧

Taos

Dusk settled in on the first night of the Molecular Mechanisms conference. Two hundred scientists, weary from travel but rejuvenated by the cold, pure mountain air, fell into their chairs to listen to Stanley Prusiner's keynote address. Perhaps he couldn't compete with Monica Lewinsky's pitiful tale, but he had prepared some drama of his own.

Prusiner had swept-back white hair, and an arched brow that conveyed authority when he spoke. He also had a surprisingly bitter tone in his voice, as though someone had taken something from him that he knew he would never get back. Though he was world-famous for his discovery of "prions"—the previously unknown infectious proteins that cause Creutzfeldt-Jakob disease in humans and bovine spongiform encephalopathy (a.k.a. "mad cow disease") in cows—the accomplishment seemed to have left an emotional scar.

For many years Prusiner had been a pariah in the scientific community, openly ridiculed for a theory many regarded as off the wall. It seemed preposterous that mere proteins could be infectious, since they weren't really alive.

Gradually, though, the evidence accrued and Prusiner was vindicated. The prion notion was so distinct from the rest of science that the distinguished American physician Lewis Thomas called it "the strangest thing in all biology." In contrast to a virus, which injects its own DNA into the host's nucleus, using the cell machinery to make copies, infectious prions require no genetic manipulation to spread. These oddly shaped proteins destabilize other nearby proteins simply by rubbing up against them, converting the neighbors into the same malignant shape. One prion transforms the next which transforms the next, creating a chain reaction that leads to what Prusiner calls a "sticky sheet" of clumpy protein. As the immune system responds by attempting to remove all the unwelcome particles, the host brain becomes a spongy mass.

As far as anyone could tell, Alzheimer's is not an infectious prion disease (though George Glenner's death from amyloidosis had caused concern). But there were enough common elements to interest Prusiner. He also seemed interested in being here in a moral capacity, as a successful fellow researcher from a nearby disease who perhaps had some lessons to share with his research cousins.

The message was embedded in his tone of resentment. As he delivered a detailed overview of his work on an overhead projector, Prusiner also retaliated against his past tormenters. He repeatedly displayed a cartoon image of a younger Stanley Prusiner (with dark hair) being squashed by a giant thumb. The thumb represented mainstream science, which kept him down because of his unconventional ideas. Prusiner finished his talk with an acrid quote from Winston Churchill:

> Men occasionally stumble across the truth, but most of them pick themselves up and hurry off as if nothing had happened.

A fitting statement from a man of politics and war, perhaps, but not a very uplifting note from a champion of scientific inquiry. Prusiner was a sore winner; it was not very becoming. But he was a winner, nonetheless, and his tale of triumph over adversity conveyed the intended message to these elite researchers: *Don't be afraid to buck the conventional wisdom; that's how scientific progress is made.*

Seventy-two of the world's most coveted ski runs were about a ten-minute drive away from the conference. Free shuttle buses waited out front on Civic Plaza Drive, with their doors wide open; eleven hundred skiable acres under a sun that famously shines 323 days a year. But with the high stakes in mind, almost everyone quietly declined, on account of what they would have had to miss; sessions were running from 8:00 A.M. to 10:00 P.M. each day, with breaks for coffee and meals.

There was so much ground to cover, including the entire human genome, with its 30,000 genes and three billion nucleotide base pairs. In the early 1990s, much of the work had shifted to molecular genetics, as researchers began to uncover genetic links to Alzheimer's all over the human genome: Chromosomes 1, 14, 19, and 21, they discovered, each have genes that can help cause Alzheimer's.

They learned that only 5 percent of Alzheimer's cases—most of them involving onset in middle age—are caused directly by a single gene. In this small minority, the disease is inherited as simply as detached earlobes or brown eyes, from just one parent's dominant gene. Anyone carrying this gene will get the disease, if they live long enough; statistically, the victims will pass the gene and the disease on to 50 percent of their children.

The cause or causes of the other 95 percent of cases were not so clear. Much emerging evidence supported a theory that the disease is "multifactorial"—caused by an unfortunate accumulation of genes and environmental factors. According to this analysis, initiating Alzheimer's disease is like pushing a school bus over a small hill: No single individual can possibly do it alone, but the right group of players coming together at the right time can make it look easy.

Making sense of such a complex landscape required an unprecedented amount of cooperation. Scientific discovery has always depended on an ever-growing scaffold of ideas and observations. But this brand of sped-up science, where data can be retrieved, analyzed quickly, and shared instantly over the Internet, required an unimaginably intricate network. The presentations in Taos—e.g., ". . . working from data on presenilin mutations published by Karen Duff in New York and Gerard Schellenberg in Seattle, and using transgenic mice supplied by Karen Hsiao in Minneapolis, we set out to . . ."—conjured up a histopathological ballet. Teams of researchers scattered around the world, constantly aware of and reacting to the movements of everyone else, were creating an improvisational dance with a startling number of graceful interchanges.

But there was also awkwardness, and discord. At the end of the first complete day, devoted almost exclusively to understanding the building blocks of the amyloid plaques, and to whether it is not the plaques but perhaps the free-floating beta-amyloid that actually does the damage, the Mayo Clinic's John Hardy, a warm and irreverent Brit with droopy eyes and an easy smile, rose to speak. He emphasized from the outset that he wasn't promising much. "Just sort of a potpourri, bits and bobs to finish off the evening.

"I've always wanted to give a talk at ten thousand feet at ten o'clock at night with four gin-and-tonics in me," he quipped to the tired group. "We'll see how it goes."

Before he got into the meat of his talk, though, he couldn't resist a poke at an absent rival. "Allen Roses isn't here, in case you haven't noticed," he said with a grin, "so I thought I'd show this slide."

The slide, entitled "Diseases Are Processes," was a wry allusion to a long-standing dispute. For several years, Hardy had been one of the leading proponents of the "amyloid cascade hypothesis," which suggested that plaques are closer to the root of Alzheimer's than tangles. According to this theory, the disease is preceded by a buildup over time of beta-amyloid, which eventually reaches a critical mass and triggers other unwanted events, including the formation of tangles. Most Alzheimer's researchers—probably some 80 percent—had come to embrace this line of thinking and had dedicated their research to some aspect of it.

Roses, director of genetics research at the pharmaceutical giant Glaxo Wellcome, dissented. He dismissed plaques as "tombstones" and "scar tissue" that are largely irrelevant to the underlying mechanisms of the disease. The "amyloid establishment," he complained, was drawing far more resources than it merited. Roses's research had led him to believe that tau—tangles—are closer to the root of the problem. In 1992, as director of the Alzheimer's program at Duke, he had made probably the most important genetic discovery to date: a variant of a gene called ApoE, located on chromosome 19 (a human cell has 46 chromosomes), that appeared to increase the risk of developing Alzheimer's by a factor of twenty. Seven years later, it was still the only verified genetic discovery related to the more common form of the disease.

Roses had felt ignored after his discovery. No one seemed interested in following up on his breakthrough research. He saw it as a classic case of herd-mentality science. The spectacular popularity of the amyloid hypothesis, he said with his famously unvarnished candor, was simply a matter of "good scientists not being able to look objectively at science, being so subjectively involved in being right and organizing posses to make sure that other people are kept from [getting the grants]—'hang these guys so they're not in the way of what we're doing.'

"It happens in this field, and I think it has really slowed therapy. The reason I say that is because these guys don't make drugs. Drug companies make drugs. And when drug companies want to start an Alzheimer's program, what do they do? They go for what's popular, for what's in the press. They say, 'Oh, here's something in *Nature.*' And if in fact 85 percent of what you see is [amyloid research], well, some drug exec without a scientific background is going to say, 'I don't know about this crazy guy Roses, who everybody says is wrong. We'll invest in amyloid.' So what happens is that the drug companies' Alzheimer's programs are actually amyloid programs, and it feeds upon itself."

Scientists can vehemently disagree and still be close friends, of course. But not John Hardy and Allen Roses. In 1991, when Hardy was still stationed in Britain, the two got into a transcontinental telephone screaming match over a paper that Hardy was about to publish.

It was not a small event. Hardy had established a link between a rare, early-onset form of the disease and a mutation on chromosome 21. The paper would be the first genetic linkage to be associated with Alzheimer's (this was before Roses's big discovery), and it included some of Roses's data as part of the proof. On the advice of a patent lawyer and because Roses had made it clear that he didn't really believe in such a link, Hardy had decided not to show the paper to Roses or offer him coauthor credit.

But then someone leaked the paper to Roses in an anonymous fax from London's Paddington Station. "I went berserk," Roses said. The imbroglio that ensued left the Alzheimer's research community polarized.

Things had simmered down somewhat since then, but the Hardy-Roses rivalry endured. "John and Allen are civil to each other," someone close to Hardy told me in Taos, "but there's no good feeling between the two." Roses was, in fact, supposed to speak at this conference, but he bowed out at the last minute. In an E-mail correspondence, Roses dismissed the Taos conference. "Most of that is academic rehash that some of our [company] people will filter," he said. "We are advancing other technologies toward a treatment. Universities do not make drugs. Governments do not make drugs. Pharmaceutical companies make drugs."

So here, at ten thousand feet, at ten o'clock at night, Hardy was poking at Roses in his absence. "Diseases are processes" was Hardy's cagey depiction of their essential disagreement: From

Hardy's point of view, Roses didn't think of Alzheimer's as an aggregation of materials and sequence of events so much as a switch turned on by a gene.

On the third night of the conference, the "tauists" got their chance. This was the stalwart minority of researchers exploring the possibility that tangles, not the plaques, were the real key to understanding Alzheimer's.

The tau (tangle) vs. amyloid (plaque) rivalry had become intense over the previous decade. "The battle is raging like the religious wars of medieval times," observed Zaven Khachaturian. "But it's good for everyone. I like to sit on the fifty-yard line and cheer."

In her talk, Virginia Lee, half of an award-winning husband-wife team from the University of Pennsylvania, playfully jabbed the predominantly amyloid crowd. "I'll give some background info for those few of you who don't understand a lot about tau," she said. Her rivals laughed.

But it was Lee's colleague Khalid Iqbal who launched the direct assault. "The amyloid cascade hypothesis has been around for almost ten years," he said, "and some of the best scientists have been working on it. But this relationship is still not understood.

"Tonight I will propose to you that we also consider an alternative hypothesis—that Alzheimer's is fundamentally a metabolic disorder. Like hypertension and coronary heart disease, Alzheimer's is a metabolic disorder of mid to old age which requires a genetic predisposition and one or more environmental factors."

Iqbal pointed out that of all the genetic mutations and environmental factors found to correspond with Alzheimer's, none are causative—none cause Alzheimer's every time. It's also important to note, he said, that the disease can arise outside of the presence of all known risk factors.

In other words, we don't know all the causes and may never know them. The causes are so many and so complex that they aren't even what matter. What matters is the common *pathway* that the disease takes after it has started. The challenge of researchers is not to stop the train just as all the cars are being assembled and put onto a track. Rather, it is to block that track after the train gets rolling but long before it gets to its destination.

The likely pathway of this disease that ends in the death of neurons, Iqbal said, is not the formation of beta-amyloid but the hyperphosphorylation of tau—the creation of tangles.

Then Iqbal delivered the sharpest blow, suggesting that amyloid may not only *not* be the problem—it may actually be a part of the solution. Amyloid, he said, seems to be not a destructive protein but a *repair* protein. Amyloid levels, he noted, go up every time there is some harm to the brain.

This was tantamount to marching into a meeting of the Federal Reserve Board and saying, "Tonight I will propose to you that inflation is not our enemy but our ally." Iqbal was lobbing grenades here. He had not come to Taos to make new friends. Prusiner, wherever he was in that large dark room, no doubt wore a narrow grin of satisfaction. Here, clearly, was a scientist not following the pack.

It all came back to Prusiner, then, and his Churchillian taunt: "Men occasionally stumble across the truth, but most of them . . ."

Was the amyloid bandwagon a classic example of "herd science," as Allen Roses and Ruth Itzhaki charged, or was it the legitimate outcome of sober investigation? This, and not any strict question of biology, was the unspoken theme of the conference. The amyloid camp seemed to have infected nearly everyone with optimism. But was that optimism sound?

The future of Alzheimer's disease would rest on the answer.

From a distance, scientific research can seem sterile, all test tubes and assays and peptides and risk factors. The Latin terminology and white lab coats create an impression of scientists as geek technicians, anti-people people who, for reasons of extreme shyness, prefer to wallow in details, crunch numbers, and deal only with objective truth. The stereotype: Scientists are smarter than the rest of us, are uncomfortable in their extreme intelligence, and find it hard to deal with others.

But close up, the view is entirely different, much more textured and colorful. The better I came to know this elite scientific group of Alzheimer's researchers, the more I understood how profoundly human their shared endeavor really was. Not far below the surface talk of microtubules and missense mutations was a culture steeped in ambition, loyalty, secrecy, warm companionship, resentment, and greed. There were real, lasting friendships here, and career-threatening antagonisms. Science turns out to be more similar to statehouse or boardroom politics than an outsider would suspect.

As I was taking it all in, one scientist at the conference quietly reminded me that there was a lot going on beneath the surface of these talks. "An important subtext of these battles," he whispered in the middle of a presentation, "is that all of these scientists have patents on their discoveries. There's a lot of money at stake."

Not just research money, but Lear Jet and beach house money. A sweeping change in U.S. law in 1980 allowed American universities and researchers to begin applying for their own patents on discoveries made with federal research dollars. Scientists were also permitted to create for-profit corporations on the side, while maintaining their publicly sponsored university research positions. "An entrepreneurial atmosphere has begun to alter the ethos of science," is how the Tufts University ethicist Sheldon Krimsky puts it. "Norms of behavior within the academic community are being modified to accommodate closer corporate ties."

For this reason, even though the scientists traveled from all around the world to speak to one another, there was also clearly much *not* being said. While this seemed to be in direct contravention of the historically open-air philosophy of all scientific inquiry, it was also conceivable that market incentives were just what ambitious researchers needed to drive themselves even harder to win this critical race.

Just before the weekend ended, I caught a telling glimpse of this invisible layer of information. One of the last to speak was Ivan Lieberburg, not a director of a university lab but head of research and development for Elan Pharmaceuticals, based in San Francisco. *Universities do not make drugs . . . pharmaceutical companies make drugs.* Lieberburg discussed, in very general terms, all the possible treatment possibilities, and then hinted at a few areas that his company is now focusing on. He apologized to the group for having to restrict his talk; for proprietary reasons, he said, there was much he could not say. But he did drop a few hints. "We're really on the threshold of a new age," he said. "I think we're coming very close to the goal line now, thanks to what many of you have done." The tone was beyond hopeful—it was celebratory.

Afterwards, as he packed up his slides, Lieberburg turned to me and said, "This was one of the most frustrating experiences I've ever had in my life, to speak to a group like this and not tell them what I know." Stay tuned, he said. Something big is coming this summer. Something very big.

Mom hasn't been feeling good the last couple days,
I wonder if her medication has something to do with it.
She takes:

Propulsid 20 milligrams, twice a day
K-Dur 20meq SA TAB, once a day
Synthroid 0.025 milligrams, once a day
Imdur 30 milligrams, once a day
Procardia XL 60 milligrams, once a day
Prilosec 20 milligrams, once a day
Aspirin 325 milligrams, once a day
Betagan eye drops, two drops for each eye, twice a day
Trinsicon/Ferocon, once a day
Paxil 30 milligrams, once a day
Neurontin 100 milligrams, once a day
Nizoral (cream), once a day
Ditropan/Oxybutynin chloride 5 milligrams, twice a day
Extra-Strength Tylenol, once a day

After sleeping for just a little bit last night, she woke up crying. She wanted us to take her to the bank. We told her it was the middle of the night—the bank was closed. She threw a fit. We told her we have cash here in the house in case she needs it. It was futile. Everything we said made no sense to her, and she made no sense to us. She went back to bed and cried. We let her cry herself to sleep.

This morning when I went to wake her for breakfast I found her pajama bottoms "hung up to dry" and she had no Depends on. It could be that she needs a change in mood medications.

—C.J.
Toledo, Ohio

Chapter 11

A WORLD OF STRULDBRUGGS

⌦

Alois Alzheimer did not get to pursue his namesake disease for very long. In 1912, just a year after publishing his first substantial paper on Alzheimer's disease and only two years after it was named for him, he accepted a new job as head of psychiatry at the University of Breslau. On the train to assume his new post, he collapsed; a case of infectious tonsillitis had developed into rheumatic fever, spreading to the kidneys, joints, and the lining of the heart. He was taken directly from the Breslau train station to the hospital. Though he eventually gained enough strength to leave the hospital, he never fully recovered. "At the conference of German Psychiatrists in 1913 I saw him," Kraepelin later recalled. "Although outwardly he appeared sprightly/active, his mood was dejected and depressed; he looked into the future with bleak foreboding. . . . In the effort to complete his duties to the full, Alzheimer did not understand how to protect himself."

Alzheimer grew weaker and weaker and finally died in 1915. He was fifty-one—the same age that his famous patient Auguste D. had been when she first experienced symptoms of forgetfulness.

For someone born in the mid–nineteenth century, fifty-one years was not brief: Life expectancy for Alzheimer's generation in Germany was somewhere in the low forties. Alois Alzheimer's boss in Frankfurt, Emil Sioli, lived to be seventy; the legendary cellular pathologist Rudolf Virchow lived to be eighty-one; but these were the exceptions. "Although historical records indicate that older people have always existed in human societies," says University of Chicago epidemiologist S. Jay Olshansky, "survival beyond age fifty for most members of a population was a rare event until the twentieth century."

Today, endurance is the norm. One in eight Americans is over sixty-five. Ninety percent of all babies born today in the developed world will live past sixty-five.

Such a dramatic expansion of life's quantity begs the question: Can we hope to match it with comparable gains in quality?

Because there were relatively few elderly at the time, it would have been impossible for Alzheimer to imagine the implications of his work. He had identified a disease that would become a serious epidemiological problem only as human populations achieved much longer life spans. Neither he nor any of the extraordinary minds in his circle could have foreseen that "this Alzheimer's disease" would in the next century emerge as *the* central public health epidemic of the industrialized world.

Perhaps it is not so bad that they couldn't see clearly into the future. If doctors in 1910 could somehow have envisioned the appalling side effects of medical progress, the agony of neurodegeneration and other diseases of deterioration experienced mostly by people who live into their seventies and beyond, they would have found this very difficult to reconcile with their work. "Modern health care permits growing numbers of people to live to advanced age under circumstances that call into question the meaning of survival," concludes Hunter College's Harry Moody.

Olshansky echoes this sentiment. "Our society is experiencing unprecedented rates of survival into older ages," he writes, "but this success has also been accompanied by a rise in frailty and disability in the general population. This is a consequence that neither the medical community nor society was prepared for."

A 1997 "State of World Health" report by the World Health Organization began this way: "Dramatic increases in life expectancy, combined with profound changes in lifestyles, will lead to global epidemics of cancer and other chronic diseases in the next two decades. The main result will be a huge increase in human suffering and disability."

Epidemiologists call this extension of frailty time a "prolongation of morbidity." It is the paradox that the extension of life inevitably yields new suffering. Alzheimer's is perhaps the perfectly poignant emblem of this medical quandary: As we defeat disease, we also create disease. Any particular illness may be conquered, but mortality is unavoidable.

Evolutionary biologists are also fascinated by the rapid increase in longevity and its unintended consequences. From their perspective, the central concept here is one of *hidden diseases*—disorders that have always existed for human beings in a potential state, but that have never been fully realized until recently.

Hidden diseases only emerge after inordinate wear and tear. A serious cyclist buying a state-of-the-art touring bicycle, for example, can expect to repair and replace many parts on a fairly predictable schedule: tires, inner tubes, and brake pads will all wear down; the bike's chain and ball bearings in the wheels' hubs will require constant lubrication, and even then they will seriously fatigue after several thousand miles. For these parts and others, replacement is common, expected, necessary.

It will take some extreme use, though—imagine crisscrossing the United States several hundred times—to wear out a set of handlebars or the bicycle's frame. There are weaknesses hidden somewhere in those durable parts that are impossible to predict and not even relevant until an extremely advanced age of use.

The long-term frailties are there somewhere, but they cannot be seen. For some fifty thousand years, as the vast majority of human beings died under the age of fifty, disorders like hearing loss, prostate cancer, osteoarthritis, breast cancer, colon cancer, amyotrophic lateral sclerosis, and Alzheimer's disease were mere diseases-in-waiting. Only in the last fifty to one hundred years have they started to come into view.

Given this, perhaps the most remarkable thing about the history of senile dementia is that it has been so conspicuous. In practical terms, it was a hidden disease with very few victims before the twentieth century, and yet references to senility are strangely ubiquitous throughout recorded history—not just in medical records, but also in legal, political, and cultural texts. Sometime around 500 B.C. the Greek legislator Solon mentioned that impaired thinking due to old age could invalidate a last will and testament. A reference to dotage is included in the "Story of the Larrikin and the Cook," one of the tales from the fifteenth-century *The Thousand and One Nights*. The *Florentine Codex,* a history of Aztec culture in Mesoamerica compiled by the Franciscan monk Bernardino de Sahagún in the sixteenth century, mentions the "childish" grandfather and other "foolish" old people. Other earlier chroniclers of senility include Euripides, Chaucer, Montaigne, Chekhov, Balzac, Carlyle, Hugo, Trollope, Conan Doyle, Bernard Shaw, Joyce, Melville, Conrad, Tocqueville, Wharton, Darwin, Cooper, Poe, Hawthorne, Sinclair Lewis, O. Henry, Sir Walter Scott, Dickens, and Thoreau. In *War and Peace,* Tolstoy wrote:

> The prince had aged very much that year. He showed marked signs of senility by a tendency to fall asleep, forgetfulness of quite recent events, remembrance of remote ones, and the childish vanity with which he accepted the role of head of the Moscow opposition.

The question is, *Why* was senile dementia such a popular topic when the sufferers were so few and its practical impact on society minimal?

In myth and fable, senility often intersects with immortality. In the Greek myth "Eos and Tithonus," Eos, goddess of the dawn, asks Zeus to grant immortality to her mortal lover Tithonus. Acting like a vindictive schoolmaster intent on teaching a lesson about linguistic precision, Zeus complies in letter but not in spirit; he bestows onto Tithonus immortality—but not eternal youth. Tithonus does live on and on, but in time becomes decrepit and senile. Eos, instead of being blessed with an endless life of passion and companionship, is consigned to the role of everlasting caregiver. Unwilling to bear the endless burden, she eventually shuts Tithonus up in a box, where he remains forever, paralyzed and babbling.

In *Gulliver's Travels,* Jonathan Swift amplified this ancient tale into the grisly spectacle of the Struldbruggs, a subrace of immortal beings born at random among the mortal Luggnaggians. When first told that these rare immortals exist—some eleven hundred of them, including fifty in the city he is currently visiting—the foreign traveler Lemuel Gulliver is gleeful. A society with immortals in its midst, he presumes, is virtually guaranteed to be enlightened—"Happy People who enjoy so many living Examples of ancient Virtue, and have Masters ready to instruct them in the Wisdom of all former Ages!" The immortal elites, he reasons, will provide the best possible insurance against the repeating of past mistakes. With a living history as its guide, civilization will inevitably become smarter and stronger.

But Gulliver has gotten it all wrong. After much laughter at his expense, the Luggnaggians politely explain that immortality, far from being a blessing, is in fact the worst imaginable curse. The actual lives of the Struldbruggs fell into this pattern:

> They commonly acted like Mortals till about Thirty Years old, after which by Degrees they grew melancholy and dejected. . . . When they came to Fourscore Years, which is reckoned the Extremity of living in this Country, they had not only all the Follies and Infirmities of other old Men, but many more which rose from the dreadful Prospect of never dying. They were not only opinionative, peevish, covetous, morose, vain, talkative; but uncapable of Friendship, and dead to all natural Affection, which never descended below their Grandchil-

dren. . . . They have no Remembrance of any thing but what they learned and observed in their Youth and middle Age, and even that is very imperfect. . . . In talking they forget the common Appellation of Things, and the Names of Persons, even of those who are their nearest Friends and Relations. For the same Reason they never can amuse themselves with reading, because their Memory will not serve to carry them from the Beginning of a Sentence to the End.

Gulliver's Travels was completed in 1725, when Swift was fifty-eight. He had long since established himself as a powerful intellect, able to wield his severe wit as a weapon against religious and political adversaries. For all of his success, though, Swift had also long exhibited a deep personal fear—a near-obsession—with the idea that his mind would slowly fade away. As a boy, he had watched in horror as his uncle Godwin withered under the forces of senility, and Swift never seemed to let go of the dark certainty that he would follow the same course. In his middle years, on a walk with the poet-clergyman Edward Young and other friends, Swift dramatically pointed to a diseased elm tree and declared, "I shall be like that tree; I shall die first at the top." He frequently complained in letters to friends about the quality and future of his memory. Swift's close friend John Boyle, the fifth Earl of Orrery, later recalled that he "heard him often lament the particular misfortune to human nature, of an utter deprivation of the senses many years before a deprivation of life." He arranged that most of his estate be devoted to the creation of a new psychiatric hospital. (Swift also complained of dizziness, nausea, and hardness of hearing all of his life, which in hindsight has been identified with some confidence as Ménière's disease, a disorder of the inner ear. Ménière's disease does not lead to memory loss or dementia.)

As he headed into his early sixties Swift's prodigious intellect was still clearly intact, but written and spoken complaints of memory loss increased. In "Verses on the Death of Dr. Swift," an autobiographical caricature written in 1731 (at age 64) about his own future demise, Swift proclaimed:

> Poor gentleman, he droops apace:
> You plainly find it in his face.
> That old vertigo in his head
> Will never leave him till he's dead.
> Besides, his memory decays;
> He recollects not what he says;
> He cannot call his friends to mind;
> Forgets the place where last he dined. . . .

Finally, as Swift approached the age of seventy, his worst fears were realized. Little by little, he began to lose his memory. Aphasia also slowly set in. He complained in one letter, "I neither read nor write, nor remember, nor converse," and in another that he could "hardly write ten lines without blunders, as you will see by the numbers of scratchings and blots before this letter is done. Into the bargain I have not one rag of memory." He became dependent on his generous cousin Martha Whiteaway as a full-time caregiver. Friends began to address their letters directly to her, and she would respond on his behalf.

Swift's decline was clearly a steady and progressive one, chiefly centered on memory. It was not, as later claimed by William Makepeace Thackeray, Samuel Johnson, and other Swift detractors, the emergence of a full-fledged, violent "lunacy" that had always been lurking in his personality. Like Cordell Annesley's oldest sister, Thackeray and Johnson sought to misappropriate the symptoms of dementia for their own purposes—in their case to diminish Swift's literary stature. History reveals their cynicism, and connects them morally with every other soul who lazily and/or greedily contorts a case of senility into some general impugning of the victim's character.

The unraveling continued. By 1740, when Swift was seventy-three, Mrs. Whiteaway reported to friends that his memory had gotten so bad he could no longer finish or correct any of his written work. Swift himself wrote in a short note to her, "I hardly understand one word that I write." Two years after that, he no longer recognized Mrs. Whiteaway and became violently abusive of her. Even with all of her affection for Swift, it was more than she could take. A housekeeper and a servant were left to care for him. A commission of friends and local officials concluded in a report in 1742 (when Swift was seventy-five) that he was "of such unsound mind and memory that he is incapable of transacting any business, or managing, conducting, or taking care either of his estate or person." In other words, he had apparently reached the middle stages of senile dementia.

It was in June of that same year that a violent and controversial episode with a local rector, Dr. Francis Wilson, marked the end of Swift's social interactions. There are differing accounts as to exactly what happened during the afternoon Swift spent with Wilson, a friend who was at that time seeking a high position at Dublin's St. Patrick's Cathedral, where Swift was dean. It is clear that Wilson came to visit Swift and persuaded him to leave his home and dine with him without the usual accompaniment of Swift's housekeeper/aide. It is also clear that Swift drank a good deal of wine and spirits at the meal and afterward—perhaps at the strong urging of Wilson. Whatever happened between the two, whether or not Wilson was loading Swift up with liquor in order to gain his endorsement for the new post, the evening ended badly.

On the way home in a carriage, Swift became enraged with Wilson and struck him. According to Wilson's account, Swift had suddenly and without provocation flown into "a most astonishing rage," cried out that Wilson was the devil, hit him, scratched him, and tried to poke his eyes out. Swift's arm was later very badly bruised. Wilson then ordered a stop to the carriage and cursed his companion. "You are a stupid old blockhead," he yelled at the severely demented Swift as he fled, "and an old rascal." Swift was taken back to his home.

By the time he got there, though, he had apparently forgotten the entire event. "Where is Dr. Wilson?" he asked his servant. "Ought not the doctor to be here this afternoon?" He could not recall even having seen him that day.

The clear intent of Swift's Struldbrugg morality play was to illustrate the same paradox that demographers would stumble onto two centuries later: *By extending our lives, we achieve suffering.* Of this Swift was certain. He also seemed to know somehow that his own demise would embody this theme. The combination of his progressive dementia and a series of unrelated and excruciating physical setbacks rendered him an almost perfect icon of wretched aging. As things got worse and worse, Lord Orrery wrote to Martha Whiteaway. "I am sorry to hear his appetite is good," he offered. "... The man I wished to live the longest, I [now] wish the soonest dead. It is the only blessing than can now befall him."

Orrery's ambivalence is now ours. It is estimated that one in nine baby boomers could live to be one hundred years old. For their grandparents' generation that figure was one in five hundred. We are in essence creating a world full of Struldbruggs, people living *en masse* into very old age and paying the consequences for it—the "rise in frailty" and prolongation of morbidity that will inevitably accompany increasing age.

Still, we pursue longevity, as individuals and as a species, and we do so without apology. It is our natural instinct to want to live, or perhaps more accurately to desperately want not to die, and to want our friends and relatives also not to die.

How will we face this new abundance of frailty: By merely trying to conquer it all, crying out in frustration whenever we fail? Or by also seeking to reconcile with the inevitable, to decline with grace, to establish a calm acceptance of our mortality? "It is time to be old/To take in sail," Emerson wrote in "Terminus." "... 'The port, well worth the cruise, is near/And every wave is charmed.'" In his diminished vista, he set out to live a life of peace and acceptance, a slow and happy fade.

In order for us to make intelligent choices about how we decline, it is important to understand why death exists in the first place. Why, indeed, are we not immortal? Is there some social or biological utility to death? Most everything in the physical world seems to have a rational basis if we look closely enough. So what is the point of dying?

In 1825, a British actuary named Benjamin Gompertz noticed

something peculiar in his mortality tables. Plotted on a graph, ages of death formed a graceful U. The probability of dying, he noticed, was very high at birth; it declined rapidly during the first year of life, and continued to decline up to the age of sexual maturity. From there it increased rapidly, exponentially even, until very old age. In sum, the older you got after birth, the less of a chance you had of dying—up until puberty, that is, at which point the older you got, the *more* of a chance you had of dying. Gompertz theorized that he had detected a hidden Law of Mortality, some sort of natural order of living and dying.

He had. Over the following two centuries, evolutionary biologists and population geneticists helped refine this law, which helped them understand the purpose of death—or, rather, its purposelessness.

Death, they came to realize, is not a part of the plan. It is not programmed into the code of life in the same way that, say, a firecracker is designed to explode. Death is also not nature's way of clearing space for future generations. Nor is it a genetic guarantee that miscreants will not be able to make trouble into eternity. Death is not nature's way of rationing energy so that the maximum number of individuals get a chance to live.

Rather, death is an unwanted but unavoidable by-product of life in the same way that a wood fire leaves us with a pile of carbon residue. The fundamental design of all life, according to the law of natural selection, is the continual adaptation of a species, *through reproduction,* to maximize long-term survival. Adaptation happens through a natural genetic variation; those variants best suited to the environment will survive the longest.

There is no particular requirement that all of these genetic variants have a built-in death spiral. It just happens that, so far, *all* of the best possible designs for a successful reproductive organism result in a structure that is highly vulnerable to deterioration some-time *after* the reproductive period. Think of a light bulb that is designed to burn very brightly; its essential purpose is its intensity, and a by-product of that intensity is that it will burn out.

A more precise analogy, one suggested by the University of Chicago's Olshansky, is the Indianapolis 500 race car, a machine designed with one very specific goal—to get to the end of that five-hundredth mile with as much speed as possible. What happens to the car in the 501st mile and every mile thereafter is of no particular concern to the designer. Every detail of design must be aimed toward the first five hundred miles. "From an evolutionary perspective," says Olshansky, "the race is to reproduction, which includes a time for the production of offspring, a possible child-rearing period, and for some species (for instance, human beings) a grandparenting period where parental contributions can be made to the reproductive success of their own offspring."

The point of the analogy is that, in designing a vehicle to go a precise distance at top speed, specific choices have to be made that favor those priorities. Those choices seem to inevitably result in long-term weaknesses that will prevent the car from lasting as long as it might have. "It is important to realize," says Olshansky, "that the cars are not intentionally engineered to fall apart—they are simply not designed to run indefinitely beyond the end of the race."

Hence Benjamin Gompertz's U-shaped mortality curve. The Law of Mortality dictates that every living organism makes reproduction a priority *at the expense of longevity.* If an individual survives the harrowing process of being born, it has a built-in maximized chance of making it to sexual potency. After that, the forces of deterioration start to overcome the forces of life.

Epidemiologists refer to the postreproductive period of life as the "genetic dustbin," because any genetic expression that occurs only in late life is simply beyond the reach of natural selection. A gene that causes a man to be very short in stature *might* help or hurt his chances to adapt to the environment and to procreate. But a gene that causes a woman's hair to turn gray when she is seventy will have no effect at all. Her genes are already passed on or not passed on, without any regard to whether that trait was a desirable one.

So-called hidden diseases, then, are hidden not just in the sense of not being visible to pre-twentieth-century human beings. More importantly, they are hidden from the forces of natural selection.

In 1998, Olshansky and his colleagues were surprised to discover something new about the Law of Mortality: that medical science had been able to *alter* it. Sorting through mortality data from mice, beagles, and humans who had died of natural causes, they were able to chart Gompertz U-shaped mortality curves in order to reveal each animal's genetic schedule of mortality—what they called their "mortality signatures." The human mortality signature turned out to be eighty-three. This means that if all of the external threats to the human body were removed, the point at which it would be most likely to simply give out averages around the age of eighty-three.

What they didn't expect, though, was a U-shaped mortality curve with a different *shape* for humans than for the other animals.

This meant that modern medicine has not only reduced external threats, but has also somehow overcome internal rhythms. "The change in rates," reported Olshansky, "indicates that the intrinsic mortality signature of human beings, something that we once thought was intractable, is being *modified.*"

We're pushing our bodies past their own innate limits. Due to extraordinary medical interventions in cancer, heart disease, and other conditions, humankind is now living longer than our genes would ordinarily allow. We are outliving our own mortality signature, living on what epidemiologists call "manufactured time." It is the cushion of extra life that we are creating for ourselves with our ingenuity and our tools.

The real challenge, of course, is to insure that this new time is something we are happy to have.

This was the second day of nearly total confusion for Ed. He was back pretending to drive the locomotives and imagining that I was one of the crew. I was asked to call the dispatcher and find out how to get back to Walla Walla.

Periodically, he asked me what Arda was doing and if I'd heard from her and telling me what a special person she is to him. (Arda is me.)

This afternoon we went for a ride, then stopped for a bite to eat. Our bill was $13.11, which Ed insisted on paying. He pulled two fifty-dollar bills out of his wallet. I told him I had the right change so I took the bill and paid it.

When we pulled up under the carport at home he said, "I'll wait here. What are we stopping here for?" He is at least cheerful and relaxed, much like a little child waiting to be told what to do. It could be worse.

—A.B.
Walla Walla, Washington

Chapter 12

HUMANIZE THE MOUSE

◦

In the 1980s, as researchers began to contemplate the possibility of trying to defeat Alzheimer's disease, the search for a fitting animal model became paramount. No one could develop a successful Alzheimer's drug without first testing it, and refining it, on animals. In order to save human lives, many thousands of nonhuman lives would first be forfeited to science. These animals would be bred according to certain desirable characteristics, kept in strictly controlled environments, examined for changes in behavior and intelligence, and ultimately sacrificed. Their brains would be taken apart, fixed in solution, sliced thinly, and examined under a microscope; or their brains would be spun in a centrifuge and analyzed chemically; or their brains would be placed in a petri dish with a variety of toxins. Collectively, these brains would serve as the proverbial drawing board onto which researchers would sketch all possible ideas for a cure.

The trouble was that, as far as anyone could tell, no other creature naturally suffers from Alzheimer's. It is a disease of sophistication. In much the same way that a bicycle cannot acquire muffler problems, animals with much less developed brains cannot experience the same sort of progressive memory loss and insidious cognitive decline as human beings.

So researchers looked for the best possible substitute, indications of a less elaborate senile dementia in lesser-developed mammals. At ten or eleven years of age, they noted, some dogs start to have sleeping trouble, pacing around at night and getting lost in familiar surroundings. When researchers took a look at their brains under the microscope, they found amyloid plaques similar to those in human Alzheimer's victims—but no tangles. They also discovered the same tangle-less pathology in cats, bears, squirrel monkeys, and lemurs.

In aging polar bears and sheep, they saw just the reverse—tangles but no plaques. No one could find a single animal, aside from humans, that had them both.

But that wasn't the biggest impediment. Ultimately, what made each of these animals unsuitable for Alzheimer's research was their longevity. Few researchers can afford to spend a decade or more waiting for a lab animal to be old enough for study.

Mice, by contrast, age quickly. They rarely live longer than two years. Mice are also easy to breed and to handle. They are by far the most popular animals for lab research. But to Alzheimer's researchers, mice were virtually useless. Very old mice displayed some slight cognitive impairment, but nothing that could be classified as dementia. Their brains accrued neither plaques nor tangles. So researchers set out to "humanize" mice—to somehow trick their bodies into acquiring a disease that evolution had spared them.

Humanizing mice was an outlandish scientific scheme. It was one thing to try to understand an animal's biology in great detail, and quite another to try and fundamentally change it—not after it was formed but during assembly. Engineers could make a car more like a train by putting it on tracks. But how could biologists change the construction of a mouse so as to make it more like a human being?

There was no way, prior to the 1980s. But then came a new technology that made humanizing not only possible but almost routine. It was called *transgenics*—the transfer of genes from one species to another.

The science of genetics dates back to the Austrian monk Gregor Mendel who, in the 1850s and 1860s, conducted hundreds of controlled breeding experiments with the garden pea *(Pisum sativum)* that proved the existence of genes. Heredity was not, Mendel demonstrated, a process of indiscriminate blending in which the traits of the parents were simply mixed together in a metaphoric vat. Rather, it was a composite of the parents' distinct genes, a mosaic of sorts.

But Mendel's work wasn't publicly recognized until 1900, sixteen years after his death. In the meantime, Charles Darwin, in 1859, introduced the broader concepts of evolution and natural selection, which were immediately catapulted into worldwide prominence. For a while, Darwin's lofty ideas levitated in the culture without essential infrastructural support, without a grounded explanation for how genetics actually works. What scientists at the time failed to realize was how volatile such intellectual instability can be. Without the nitty-gritty Mendelian details, Darwinism was left vulnerable to misunderstanding and manipulation.

One extremely dangerous misconception was the notion of "degeneration," introduced by psychiatrist and theology student Augustin Morel. Morel reasoned that if evolution helped the fittest rise to the top, it must also actively push the least fit to the bottom. Undesirable traits would not merely be passed over; they would grow less and less desirable with each successive generation. The hook nose of the parent would become more hooked in the child, the cleft palate more cleft, the low intelligence even lower. Character traits and morals would be passed on and amplified in the same way. Morel wrote:

> This deviation even if, at the outset, it was ever so slight, contained transmissible elements of such a nature that [the patient] becomes more and more incapable of fulfilling his functions in the world; and mental progress, already checked in his own person, finds itself menaced also in his descendants.

The traits from one generation would get worse in the next; the entire family line would *degenerate*. In effect, Morel proposed that undesirable genetic traits—and their human carriers—were themselves diseases. The health of human society depended on the eradication of these diseased genes.

It was a perverse, wrongheaded proposal, made in ignorance and with the hubris that science could serve humanity by destroying many humans. But in the pre-Mendelian vacuum, many scientists found degeneration theory irresistible. All over Europe, doctors rushed to create lists of physical and mental deformities that indicated a degenerative spiral in a particular family or group.

In Germany, the Society for Racial Hygiene was formed in 1905 as a way of defending civilization against genetic impurities. Emil Kraepelin and Alois Alzheimer both joined. Though not overtly racist in its conception, degeneration theory helped to nudge German society down a slippery slope toward ethnic bias and xenophobia of all nonconforming individuals and groups.

At the bottom of that slope: Hitler's Final Solution, the systematic extermination of Jews, Gypsies, homosexuals, the handicapped, the mentally ill, and others considered degenerate. "We may—and we must—rely on the healthy instincts of the best of our people," zoologist Konrad Lorenz wrote in 1940 to support Nazi aims, "for the extermination of elements of the population loaded with dregs. Otherwise, these deleterious mutations will permeate the body of the people like the cells of a cancer."

Alois Alzheimer, whose wife came from a prominent Jewish family, was not a proto-fascist. Though he was receptive to the notion of degeneration, he was also wary of its social implications. "Perhaps the future," he wrote, "will let us see more clearly here and then show other principles to advantage; today we would go on interminably, if we were to see ourselves as justified in placing into the balance the inferiority of the descendants of the mentally ill, when we have to decide whether a termination of pregnancy is appropriate or not." In a 1999 biography of Alzheimer, Konrad Maurer wrote, "With that [remark], Alzheimer distinguished himself very clearly, and very early on from his colleagues [Alfred Friedrich] Hoche and [Ernst] Ruedin, who would later provide the weaponry for a terrible development."

Science as weaponry: the metaphor is a reminder of scientists' awesome power. The naming of diseases is a powerful social act that in turn can dictate social behavior. It therefore behooves the public to keep a close watch over the definition of diseases, of the power of doctors to decide what is and is not a part of healthy human society. Like the military, the scientific establishment should ultimately be under the watch of civilians ensuring the public will.

In 1953, James Watson and Francis Crick proposed the double-helix model as the structure of DNA, a spiral-shaped chain of deoxyribonucleic acid molecules that contained programming information for the function of all living organisms. In the following decades researchers began to construct a crude map associating particular genes with specific functions and diseases. By the 1980s, scientists could not only analyze the sequence of DNA strands but, incredibly, could also chemically remove—"knock out"—a tiny snippet and insert a replacement. When they had honed the technique enough to do this inside a just-fertilized mouse egg, the first humanized mouse was born. So-called knock-out mice became a powerful new tool for researchers all across the disease spectrum.

Nature may favor survival of the fittest, but with their startling new power, geneticists often found themselves working in the other direction—toward a degeneration of their own making. Commonly, knock-out technology was used to proliferate flawed genes—what Konrad Lorenz called the *dregs*—for closer study. Instead of building a "better mousetrap," as the business cliché goes, they created worse mice: artificially obese mice, diabetic mice, deaf mice, muscular dystrophy mice, Huntington's disease mice, asthmatic mice, cystic fibrosis mice, cancer mice, heart disease mice, and—in 1996—Alzheimer's mice.

Or at least the first reasonably close approximation. By splicing in a human gene that causes harmless APP to dissolve into sticky beta-amyloid, the University of Minnesota's Karen Hsiao created the first mouse with plaques. The descendants of this humanized mouse appeared normal at birth. But at nine or ten months, they started having considerable memory trouble. In a pool of water, they would lose the ability to learn and remember the location of a platform. In dry mazes, they kept forgetting where the exits were. It was about as close to Alzheimer's disease as researchers could imagine in a mouse. When Hsiao opened up their brains, she saw that they were filled with amyloid plaques. It was a major breakthrough.

Of course, not everyone liked the idea of inflicting human diseases on animals. In 1999, animal rights activists broke into several University of Minnesota labs. They took forty-eight mice—including several of Hsiao's—along with thirty-six rats, twenty-seven pigeons, and five salamanders, and destroyed lab equipment worth several million dollars. They also spray-painted walls with slogans such as "No More Torture" and complained of electrodes being attached to animals' heads.

Five of the "liberated" animals were found dead the next day in a nearby field. Meanwhile, university scientists effectively refuted the activists' claims: The electrodes were not a part of some shock treatments, but harmless measurement devices, the same as those used to measure brain waves on humans. By no means were these animals being "tortured." To the contrary, lab animals all across the country were now protected by an elaborate legal and ethical regimen that guaranteed them a hygienic, nutritious, and pain-free environment. For reasons of liability, personal conscience, and good science, modern researchers generally treated their animals well and sacrificed only as many as were necessary.

Still, lab animals were being held against their will, drugged, and killed. The relatively humane treatment of the animals did not address the most basic charge of animal rights activists: that it is immoral to sacrifice animals merely to improve the health of human beings. To their credit, many modern researchers seem ready to address the issue head-on. "I am sure that we do have such duties to behave kindly and with respect to other animals, with the minimum of violence and cruelty, not to damage or take their lives insofar as it can be avoided," writes British neurobiologist Steven Rose. ". . . [B]ut all such duties to nonhuman animals are limited by an overriding duty to other humans." If sacrificing these animals can reduce human suffering, most researchers strongly believe, it is morally necessary. Their duty is not to the preservation of life in general, but human life in particular.

Despite protests, overall public sentiment and market economics strongly supported transgenics, and it flourished. By 1998, more than 500,000 transgenic mice were being used annually in experiments across the research spectrum. The technology was a critical breakthrough for Alzheimer's research in particular, finally giving scientists a reliable animal model. Dozens of variant strains followed from the original Hsiao knock-off Alzheimer's mouse and became the basis of many important Alzheimer's breakthroughs in the late 1990s.

The marketplace not only encouraged the creation of these

mice; it also insisted on their commodification. Not long after the Taos conference, Elan Pharmaceuticals—the company promising a dramatic development "very soon"—instead slammed the community with litigation. The company filed suit against the nonprofit Mayo Foundation for selling a strain of Hsiao mice on which Elan claimed to hold a patent.

The lawsuit hit the field like a cluster bomb, with subpoenas hitting other researchers all over who were working with knock-out mice created on the Hsiao model. Elan demanded to see the contents of their lab notebooks. "It's outrageous," remarked Karen Duff of the Nathan Kline Institute. Johns Hopkins microbiologist David Borchelt insisted that he would go to jail before turning his notebooks over to Elan.

The Mayo Clinic's Steven Younkin lashed out at Elan by contrasting the company's ethic with that of the mouse's original "inventor," Karen Hsiao. "Karen decided on Day One that she was giving her mouse to any academic researcher who asked for it," he said. "I think [Elan's] strategy is, 'Let's make sure we make all the money we possibly can, and if it slows down research, that's too bad. We've got our shareholders to worry about.'"

The notion of scientists fighting in court for the exclusive right to create a defective mouse was grotesque. But the new genetics lent itself to such absurdity, since it gave humans the power to alter the basic building blocks of life. In pursuit of their own interests, corporate managers saw little choice but to reduce transgenic creations to matters of contract and property law. The irony of the effort to "humanize" these mice, then, was that they were also simultaneously pushed in a very different direction—out of the realm of living beings entirely. It is as though the mice, now that they were programmable, were nothing more than machinery.

A California judge dismissed the Elan lawsuit, ruling that the company's patent was invalid. Officials from Elan declined to make any public comment on the case, other than to say that it was "Elan's policy to enforce its intellectual property rights," and that in the wake of the court dismissal the company was continuing to examine its legal options. Its litigiousness reflected the changing climate in science, a lurch toward the free market that gave primacy to making money rather than sharing information. Since 1980, when Congress significantly loosened restrictions on the interaction between public and private research efforts, many academic researchers had taken personal investment stakes in their own research. A 1996 survey of articles in leading U.S. biomedical journals revealed that close to one-third of the lead authors had some significant financial interest in the issues discussed in their published report.

Overall, the community was ambivalent about the new opportunities to benefit financially from their own research. "It brings out the worst in some people," said Glaxo Wellcome's Allen Roses. "And there is no field as bad as Alzheimer's. I've been in several fields including muscular dystrophy and human genetics, which is known to be bad because things can be so easily stolen, but Alzheimer's disease is the epitome of this because there's so much money at stake."

But Roses also had much to say in favor of the marketization of science. From where he sat, it was clearly faster and more efficient. Just two years after leaving Duke University for his new corporate post, he had already pioneered the use of a new technology called "SNP mapping." SNP, pronounced "snip," stands for single nucleotide polymorphisms, single-molecule variations in human DNA that determine whether someone is susceptible to a certain disease or would be responsive to a certain drug. SNP mapping helps to narrow substantially the search for disease genes by reducing the amount of information that needs to be analyzed—the equivalent of telling a researcher at the Library of Congress that instead of having to search randomly through the open stacks for a particular book by Kurt Vonnegut, he can instead check the card catalogue file under "Von." "In diabetes," Roses cited as an example, "we can go from 50 million base pairs down to ten thousand."

Because his discovery was privately funded, Roses openly bragged, he was not bound to share anything about it until after the money is in the bank. "One of the things we want to do before we release it," he said about one SNP development, "is get the functional genomic mice we need ready to go. That way, we're way far ahead and it's very expensive for anybody to try and catch up—like when Duke is ahead of its opponent and the students turn their back and scream, 'It simply doesn't matter.' " He laughed.

This was the new scientific ethic, as dictated by corporate managers: *Get products to market.* In his former academic life, Roses had spent decades applying for government grants, publishing in prestigious journals, and attending a whirlwind of academic conferences. He no longer did any of this—not just because he didn't have to, he said, but also because he was convinced that academic science had become permanently corrupted by money, and that he had found a new and much better way. As an academic, Roses said, he merely fought over ideas. As a corporate pharmacogeneticist, he was actually working to conquer diseases.

"I was in a situation where I was spending 50 to 60 percent of my time writing grants that never got funded," he said of the contrast. "We argued for three years about whether ApoE is inside neurons or not. It is in the neurons. We went to every meeting. They said, 'It's not in the neurons.' We would write a grant proposal. 'Oh, you can't do that—it isn't in neurons.' No grant. So what we have now done is say, 'Piss off. We're just going to do it. We're going to do it right and objectively, on the basis of the data.' I can tell you, we have found differences in the brain metabolism in these mice where the only difference is ApoE3 versus ApoE4. What they are and how we target them—I don't have to publish that. I don't have to take the time or the people it would involve to publish it.

"Am I keeping anything from my fellow researchers around the world in Alzheimer's disease? Hell no! All they ever did when I ever said anything was to say, 'No, no, no.' We would just argue it at all these scientific meetings. Now we debate in the context of very critical, highly skilled scientists who know that our viability as a team, our viability as a company, and our jobs depend on it—not whether we get it first into publication."

In fact, Roses *was* withholding information, as he acknowledged. His point seemed obvious. He was arguing that, in the new context of market science, withholding information was more efficient. The ends justified the means. The market would sort things out.

Mother has for some time referred to herself in the third person. Usually this happens when we have been talking about her for a little while. She will ask a question that fits right in to the conversation, but begins, "Does she . . ." If I ask to whom she is referring, she'll answer, "That woman we have been talking about."

There are also lots of double people here. My husband is "the boys." My daughter's friend, who came over so I could go to a support group, was just one person when she walked out the door, but within fifteen minutes was two! I am a different person in the morning, afternoon, and night, which is logical considering that she thinks she's living (and working) in an institution. She was a nurse, so three shifts, right? Sometimes I'm different within the hour: "I can't go to the store with you because that other girl is taking me somewhere else."

—M.A.J.
Nampa, Idaho

Chapter 13

WE HOPE TO RADIO BACK TO EARTH
IMAGES OF BEAUTY NEVER SEEN

◦

In a short story by Jorge Luis Borges, a group of elite mapmakers are given an inherently unrealizable task: to create a map of the empire that is on the same scale as the empire—a map as big as its subject matter. Analogous is the challenge Morris Friedell took upon himself after receiving his Alzheimer's diagnosis. He wanted to unravel the mystery of a brain disease just as this disease was unraveling *him.* He wanted to study his own undoing.

In a sense, he'd been preparing for this project for most of his life. His college courses focused on human dignity and what he called the "social psychology of affliction." Now, in his unexpected new role among the afflicted, he could test the practicality of his ideas.

Shortly after his diagnosis he wrote a short essay entitled "Introduction to Myself and My Plight." The essay concluded:

I hope to be able to contribute to existential philosophy from a unique perspective. Perhaps, as my selfhood diminishes, I can add to the general human understanding of matters such as "self" and "time" and "nothingness." With this orientation I can perhaps make my slow dying a final intellectual and esthetic adventure.

When I was in my early teens in the 1950s I avidly read science fiction by Robert Heinlein and Arthur C. Clarke. I fantasized being an "astrogator." We collide with an asteroid, there is not enough fuel to get back to earth. We turn the ship straight away from the sun, we voyage out beyond the orbit of Pluto. We know we will perish in the interstellar void, yet we hope to radio back to earth images of beauty never seen as well as valuable information. . . . On August 19, 1998, my neurologist told me [Alzheimer's] is what the PET scan indicated. And here I am on that spaceship.

It wasn't long before he sent back his first dispatch, about a surprising advantage he discovered in forgetting. With less of a grip on what happened two hours or ten minutes ago, Morris reported feeling dramatically more involved in the present. "I find myself more visually sensitive," he said. "Everything seems richer: lines, planes, contrast. It is a wonderful compensation. . . . We [who have Alzheimer's disease] can appreciate clouds, leaves, flowers as we never did before. . . . as the poet Theodore Roethke put it, 'In a dark time the eye begins to see.'

"So many of us go through life like tourists with a camera always between our eyes and the world," Morris observed. Alzheimer's won't allow that sort of detachment. Like H.M. from the 1950s, the short-circuiting of memory forces every Alzheimer's sufferer to be always in the Now. This is widely regarded as one of the horrors of the disease. But from his firsthand experience, Morris argued that being perpetually in the Now has an upside. It leads to an actual *heightening* of consciousness. "I can watch kittens playing in a way I couldn't before," he said.

How could a neurological disease enrich awareness?

All of waking life is a stew of familiar and unfamiliar experiences; it is the brain's job to turn the unfamiliar into the familiar. Familiar sights, sounds, and ideas don't demand as much energy or attention, and can elicit quicker and more graceful responses. Thanks to familiarity, a person can do many things at once, and even process relatively complex ideas almost completely in the background, without having to bother the conscious mind.

New experiences, by contrast, demand conscious attention, so that they may be examined, understood, contextualized, reacted to, memorized, *learned.* Think of learning to play the piano or to ride a bike; think of the first time you went to a baseball game or ate sushi. The unfamiliar demands focus, greedily occupies consciousness. Confronting the new is a captivating, exhausting experience.

Alzheimer's keeps things new. After onset, the unfamiliar can never become familiar. The Alzheimer's mind is constantly flooded with new stimuli; everything is always in the moment, a rich, resonant, overwhelming feeling. "I've noticed that I have a large amount of appreciation for whatever I'm focused on," commented fellow Alzheimer's sufferer Laura S. in response to Morris's declaration. "It is very clear and real. Look away and it is gone. Look back and it is fresh and new. I am checking this out with a red geranium blossom right now. When I look away, 'red' no longer exists except as an abstract term. No blossom image remains. . . . But I can look again."

Ever-freshness, then, may be considered an Alzheimer's consolation prize. This may be a particularly difficult idea for caregivers to swallow because their own experience is often precisely the opposite. As their forgetful loved ones repeatedly stumble over the same tasks and information, caregivers must suffer through the oppressive repetition. They repeat the same mind-numbing instructions over and over again. Life threatens to become less and less fresh in the way that a tour guide quickly loses any real enthusiasm and interest in the material that she must repeat twelve times a day, five days a week. In the often deadening, disheartening world of Alzheimer's care, caregivers wake up thousands of days in a row facing the same tourist wanting to take exactly the same tour.

Still, caregivers must try to understand both the frustrations and the unexpected benefits of having an unraveling mind. What they may at first presume to be a uniformly awful experience for the victims can sometimes perhaps be peculiarly satisfying and even enriching—"a final intellectual and esthetic adventure."

In the late 1970s, close friends of the master Abstract Expressionist painter Willem de Kooning began to notice that he was having trouble remembering names and recent events, and following the thread of conversations. At the time, de Kooning was trying to escape from a decades-long dependence on alcohol, and the memory problems were assumed to be acute side effects of his difficult recovery.

It turned out that the forgetting was not the end of his alcoholism; it was the beginning of his Alzheimer's disease. He recovered his strength and, with the aid of friends, family, and a drug called Antabuse—which nauseated him every time he tasted alcohol—managed to stay on the wagon. But his forgetfulness grew steadily worse. Slowly, over nearly two decades, he unraveled entirely. His estranged wife, Elaine, who came back into his life in 1978 and became the chief architect of his recovery from alcoholism, eerily predicted the course of his later years in a frank lecture she gave him that same year.

"Bill," she said. "Your genes are sensational. Your mother lived to be ninety-two and was strong as a rock. Your father lived to eighty-nine, your grandmother to ninety-five. So your body's going to last, but your brain is going to go. You will be a vegetable."

"You're scaring me," de Kooning replied.

"Good," said his wife.

By 1983, five years later, he was forgetting so much that he started to experience moments of genuine confusion. On a transatlantic flight from New York to Amsterdam that year, de Kooning turned to Elaine in the middle of the in-flight movie and said, "This is a lousy film. Let's get out of here."

When his wife gently reminded him they were not in a New York cinema but on a plane to Europe, de Kooning revealed an even deeper confusion. "This is terrible," he said. "They'll find out I left the U.S., and they'll never let me back in again." De Kooning had originally come to the U.S. as a stowaway in 1926, and had not become an American citizen until 1961. Now, on the plane to Amsterdam in 1983, he was stuck in an old awareness, a sense of himself that had long since expired.

Such a time regression is common for Alzheimer's sufferers in the confusional stages; quite often, they find themselves jerked back so forcefully to earlier memories that they expect spouses to be young and parents to still be alive. They might also think of themselves as younger looking, failing to recognize their own faces in the mirror. All of this happens because relatively fragile memories from recent years have dissolved, leaving only much older, more durable memories. While a memory formed forty years ago is not inherently more resilient than one formed four years ago, older memories of childhood playhouses and wedding vows have become more durable through thousands of recollections in the intervening years. Since the act of remembering itself creates a brand-new memory of that memory, the most powerful images from childhood and early adulthood get replayed over and over again in a person's mind and thus become virtually indestructible by the time a person reaches his seventies. Those seasoned memories are as durable as limestone, while the more recent are still relative impressions in sand.

De Kooning, remarkably, kept painting. In fact, as he recovered from his drinking problem, he commenced in 1981 what would turn out to be one of the most productive, if also controversial, periods of his career. De Kooning not only produced an extraordinary 341 paintings over a ten-year period, but created work that has since received high critical praise—even given the general awareness of his dementia.

The paintings from the 1980s are, in many respects, very different from his earlier work. They are more melodious, graceful, and far less dense. Overall, they seem happier, far less angst-ridden, than his more famous creations. In contrast to his previously complex color palette, premixed with great care, de Kooning came to rely heavily on primary colors pulled straight out of the tube. In contrast to his thickly layered paintings from before, these late works have a lot less texture. The strokes are less animated, more relaxed; the dominant form is a bright, ribbonlike weave vaguely suggesting human curves and natural landscapes. Blank space takes a more prominent role in these late paintings—"like a blank mind picturing itself," observed art journalist Kay Larson.

"There is no question in my mind that it's an extraordinary body of work," San Francisco Museum of Modern Art curator Gary Garrels told Larson in 1994 as he organized a major exhibition of the eighties work. "There is intense concentration and consciousness in these paintings. They are not just someone spreading paint around. This is definitely an artist in control." Garrels went on further to say that many of de Kooning's works from this period are "among the most beautiful, sensual, and exuberant abstract works by any modern painter."

Critics took special notice of the 1995 Garrels exhibition because they had, by 1980, more or less written de Kooning's artistic obituary—one which included an especially unflattering final chapter. "Anyone who remembers the [1983] Whitney [retrospective] exhibition knows there are acres of sloppy, slack, fizzled paintings from the sixties and seventies," wrote Larson. "Nobody had a reason to think the eighties would be different."

But this new work, everyone agreed, *was* very different from previous periods. "The effect they gave was one of lightness and joy," Curtis Bill Pepper wrote in the *New York Times* after seeing a collection of de Kooning's latest paintings in the early 1980s. "It was an old man's lyrical elegy distilled from the turbulent recesses of the self."

Pepper did not mention that a metabolic process in de Kooning's cerebral cortex was radically redefining his "self." What was taking place in that Long Island studio was much more than a personal resurgence; de Kooning was documenting on canvas his own progressive forgetting.

Was he really a happier man? It's entirely possible. Alzheimer's can be severely frustrating to patients at certain periods, but can also leave its victims extraordinarily serene. The patient loses the awareness of what he has lost. He has fewer thoughts, fewer worries. Life is not as complex or demanding. In this sense, Emerson was speaking hopefully on behalf of all Alzheimer's sufferers when he said, "Things that go wrong . . . don't disturb me," and "I have lost my mental faculties but am perfectly well."

When, in the 1990s, the art community finally got to see the eighties work as a whole, now very aware of de Kooning's slide into dementia, there was a flood of interest in the paintings and curiosity about what they meant. Inevitably, a debate ensued about their artistry, their importance, and their connection to the artist's previous work. Ultimately, these were subjective judgments, of course, but it was only natural to wonder if de Kooning had maintained his greatness throughout illness. Were his late works genuinely a part of the *oeuvre* of one of the most important painters in the twentieth century, or should they instead be thought of as works by a once-great artist now "on autopilot," without any fresh ideas or even any ideas at all?

This was not just an academic question. Millions of dollars and the reputations of many collectors, curators, gallery owners, and critics were riding on the answer. The stakes were so high that in 1995 the San Francisco MOMA's Garrels assembled a panel that included the painter Jasper Johns and directors of several major modern art museums. (De Kooning was in the final stages of his illness at the time, no longer painting; he died in 1997.) Over two days, they reviewed and discussed scores of the late paintings, and considered some fundamental questions:

Should current works be judged as a group or individually?

Should they be judged purely on their own merits or in comparison to prior work? If the latter, how much familiarity with de Kooning's past was necessary to make sound appraisals of this work?

Should the viewer's own expectations play a role?

Should de Kooning's intentions be taken into account? If so, how could one best discern his intentions?

These were all formal and polite ways of poking at a very uncomfortable question: Could this new direction of work legitimately be seen as an extension of de Kooning's provocative career, or had he lost his artistic spark along with his functioning hippocampus? It is an impossible question to answer fully, of course, but still one well worth asking. The insidious creep of Alzheimer's erases the self in such tiny increments that trying to determine any sort of distinct cutoff point approaches the paradoxical quality of a Zen koan. What is the sound of fewer neurons firing?

One factor in sizing up the effect of Alzheimer's on the artistic process is the distinction between *mind memory* and *muscle memory*. Mind memories are formed in association between the hippocampus and the cerebral cortex, stored in the cortex, and are highly vulnerable to suggestion, to the vagaries of time, and to the plaques and tangles of Alzheimer's disease.

Muscle memory, also called *procedural memory*, exists as an entirely separate neural network in different regions of the brain. These are the unconscious, but exquisitely detailed, movements that a person makes when walking down the stairs, riding a bike, playing the piano, typing, clapping, painting, kissing. Muscle memories are much harder to lay down than mind memories—they take practice, practice, practice. But once ingrained, they are also far more difficult to erase. Notice that even victims of extreme amnesia do not "forget" how to walk. It takes a stroke or some other traumatic brain injury for muscle memories to be disrupted. Doctors were interested to discover that H.M., whose ability to form new mind memories was immediately and forever removed along with his hippocampus, could in fact develop new coordination skills—even though he was never actually aware of the new skills he had.

In the same way as H.M., Alzheimer's sufferers generally retain complete muscle memories until the very late stages of the disease, when the plaques and tangles finally creep into virtually every area of the brain. This steady erosion of intellectual capacity without noticeable physical disruption is what sparks public fascination with the disease in the first place, and haunts even the most seasoned observers. Even for people who spend years immersed in the culture of the disease, it is positively ghostly to be in the presence of a man who for several years has not recognized his wife but who can still walk or sing or even dance a waltz.

Or paint. We know, both from firsthand reports of de Kooning's studio assistants and from the closely studied patterns of Alzheimer's disease, that de Kooning's signature brushstroke did not erode at the same time that he had trouble remembering what he had eaten for breakfast. His muscle memory remained intact for a long while, and the act of painting remained important to him. People who spent time with him during his long period of forgetting say that his sagging posture and lethargic manner abruptly shifted into an erect, energetic, passionate professionalism whenever he walked from his kitchen to his adjacent studio.

What was ebbing slowly in de Kooning's brain was a refined cognition and a capacity for lucid discourse. He could no longer manage his practical affairs, engage in sophisticated conversation, or socialize on any significant level. Many years before he was forced to stop painting, he became effectively cut off from the world around him, losing the ability to discuss his work intelligently or consider it in the larger context of society and art history.

From a certain creative standpoint, such forfeitures might not be considered a liability. After all, artists are not analysts. To the contrary: Every creator knows that thinking can disrupt creativity. "Art . . . is not cognitive," Israel Scheffler wrote in his book *Symbolic Worlds,* "but rather emotive in its import. Its function is to stimulate, express, or vent emotions rather than describe reality."

Throughout his long career, de Kooning had not relied on elaborate conceptualization in the same way, for example, that Andy Warhol had to create his Campbell Soup silk screens or Georges Seurat had to create his painstaking pointillist *Sunday Afternoon on the Island of La Grande Jatte.* "De Kooning was never a very intellectual painter," wrote Kay Larson. "Even in the beginning, in the *Women* [series], in *Excavation,* his talents emerged from the moment—from the thrust and parry of the brush, from the 'excavation' of his emotional state."

One essential component of self that Alzheimer's patients do *not* come untethered from early on is their own emotional reservoir. From this vantage, it almost seems as though de Kooning contracted just the right disease, the one neurological disorder that would spare his ability to create as it ate away at most of the rest of his abilities.

Perhaps, then, Alzheimer's did not dim de Kooning's art, at least not until much later in the disease. Perhaps Alzheimer's *enhanced* his art. Morris Friedell's observation about the heightening of consciousness in the early stages of Alzheimer's would seem to apply perfectly to de Kooning and other abstract artists. If Abstract Expressionism exists predominantly as an emotional response to the world, the new freshness of consciousness forced upon early-stage Alzheimer patients could presumably serve as a creative impulse.

De Kooning himself had complained in the mid-seventies (pre-Alzheimer's) that his way of working had become "almost a habit," and critics seemed to agree wholeheartedly. It seems more than a mere coincidence that his art was rejuvenated at precisely the same time he began to succumb to the disease—to lose his ability to follow habits. One reasonable analysis is that the disruption of memories fortuitously dissolved chronic work patterns that had become such a burden. In this way, the disease may have, if only temporarily, *rescued* de Kooning's career, granting him an extra few years of creative energy by releasing him from a tired routine.

"Collectively, the pictures . . . seem to glow with an inner light," the *San Francisco Examiner's* David Bonetti wrote of de Kooning's late work. ". . . They remind you that even during bleak times, art can offer emotional and spiritual solace like nothing else." Kay Larson, writing in the *Village Voice,* pared the rejuvenation theory down to its perfect reductionist epithet: De Kooning, she wrote, rounded out his career in a fertile period of "Alzheimer's Expressionism."

One does not, of course, want to exaggerate the advantages of a slide toward oblivion. Many important faculties are, in fact, adversely affected early on in Alzheimer's: constructional abilities, spatial relations, orientation, perspective, and concentration. So even as an abstractionist, de Kooning would have had a somewhat reduced command of his craft after the onset of Alzheimer's. His ability to execute a desired stroke would in certain ways have been compromised.

Another important consideration is the impairment of so-called executive function skills, including goal-setting and self-evaluation. A person's introspection begins to wither away from near the beginning of Alzheimer's—the constant "How-am-I-doing?" inner dialogue that people with functioning brains take for granted. When introspection begins to break down, so does willfulness—"Here's-what-I-should-do-next." As the plaques and tangles proliferate and the brain begins to shrink, a psychic barrier arises between the victim and the outside world. The Alzheimer's sufferer becomes an island.

In that isolation, argue some, de Kooning's art in particular vanished completely. "Art, in the way that de Kooning conceived it, is something that is produced in a conscious dialogue with the rest of art history and culture," argues art historian András Szántó. "De Kooning is an excellent example of what we call the 'professional artist,' one who worked strictly within the context of other art. His was actually a very conceptual, aesthetic agenda, turning the art world upside down, demolishing certain assumptions that were in place up to the 1960s.

"If, later on in life, we end up with someone who is merely doing things in his head, then de Kooning's art, as he understood it, is gone. Once the dialogue with the rest of the world is severed, it is impossible to speak of this as art with a capital 'A.' "

Amidst stark disagreements about the quality of de Kooning's eighties paintings, the 1995 panel did not manage to come to a real consensus. "No single point of view predominated," Garrels politely reported, except for the agreement that the works produced after 1989 could not be counted as "fully realized works of art." Some panel members felt that the work had lost its essential structure in the mid-1980s—which is roughly when de Kooning passed into the middle stages of the disease. But others agreed with Garrels and MOMA curator Robert Storr that the work up to 1989 stands on its own.

A year after the panel deliberated, the neurologist Carlos Hugo Espinel published an essay about de Kooning in the British medical journal *Lancet.* "These paintings [are] not merely the product of someone who had simply retained colour perception and the motor strength to copy," Espinel wrote. "Even if at times he confused his wife with his sister . . . De Kooning went on to create. His resurgence is a testimony to the potential of the human mind, evidence for hope."

And there *was* hope—not that de Kooning might somehow recover from his forgetting, but that he could live serenely within it; that we could all live in harmony with the specter of senile dementia.

De Kooning was, after all, speaking for all of us, and to us. He had spent his long life producing abstract emotional pastiches, painting images from his psyche in the same way that radio announcers would depict a boxing match: in quick, emotional bursts that said something very personal about the artist and, often, also something profound about the human condition. "I am always in the picture somewhere," he said in 1950. ". . . I seem to move around in it, and there seems to be a time when I lose sight of what I wanted to do, and then I am out of it. If the picture has a countenance, I keep it. If it hasn't, I throw it away."

In these late paintings, de Kooning was presenting one final series of communiqués to his public, messages of tranquillity and transcendence in decline. It was a message that Emerson, Shakespeare, Erasmus, and others had sent: Senility, while devastating, is also a part of life.

In his essay, Espinel also briefly alluded to a feature in the late-period de Koonings that every other observer had missed: the unmistakable resemblance between the wispy strokes on his canvases and the neurofibrillary tangles in his brain.

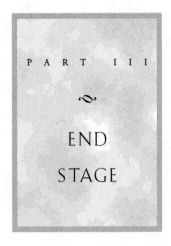

PART III

END
STAGE

Chapter 14

BREAKTHROUGH?

◦

San Francisco, California: July 1999

In July, with patents filed and publication pending, Elan Pharmaceuticals finally broke their long silence: They had a new drug that had *eliminated* plaques in mice. In the next few months they would begin testing it in humans.

The news caught researchers completely by surprise.

"It's wild and amazing," said Sangram Sisodia, chairman of neurobiology at the University of Chicago.

"This is a major step forward," said the National Institute on Aging's Marcelle Morrison-Bogorad.

Even officials from the famously cautious Alzheimer's Association gushed. "It's a fascinating finding with immense potential," offered Vice President Bill Thies. This was the first time in the organization's twenty-year history that it had issued an unqualified statement of optimism about a potential treatment.

The most surprising part of the news was the type of drug: a simple antibody vaccine, no different in principle from the vaccines for polio, measles, mumps, and diphtheria. Those vaccines work by injecting weakened bits of live virus into the bloodstream, stimulating the immune system to develop specific antibodies that quickly recognize and remove any future virus to come along.

Antibodies are not limited to virus removal; they can theoretically be programmed to tag and remove any foreign object—beta-amyloid, for instance, the main component of plaques. Beta-amyloid is just as foreign to the human body as any virus. Elan's new approach was to inject bits of beta-amyloid into the bloodstream the same way that Albert Sabin injected weakened polio virus.

It seemed like one of those ideas that was too simple to work, so much so that when lead researcher Dale Schenk had first mentioned the concept to coworkers in a brainstorming session a few years earlier, he said, "Everyone looked at me like I was crazy." The notion seemed dead on utterance; as a demonstration of its apparent absurdity, one of Schenk's colleagues pinned it to an office bulletin board of outrageous comments.

Now, other Alzheimer's researchers were admitting they would have had the same reaction. "If someone had suggested that experiment to me," said the Mayo Clinic's John Hardy after the breakthrough announcement, "I would have told them not to waste their time."

Chicago's Sisodia said: "I wouldn't have imagined it could ever work. We haven't even *thought* about a vaccine for Alzheimer's."

But to Schenk, his self-described "nutty idea" was the natural outcome of tracing what he already knew about plaques through a number of logical steps. "The absolute levels of production of beta-amyloid in the brain tissue seem to be a critical factor in whether or not you get amyloid plaques," he explained. "So I was thinking about that one day, and I thought, 'If there was only a way to tie up that beta-amyloid in the brain, to keep it occupied.' Then I thought, 'Well, maybe if we had antibodies there, that would work. It's too bad that there are no good ways to get antibodies into the brain. You could inject them straight into the brain, but that's not a good idea. . . .'

"And then it suddenly hit me like a stone: Actually, we could put antibodies into the *bloodstream,* and a small amount would likely leak into the brain. Furthermore, why don't we just immunize with beta-amyloid? Then the body would be constantly making a ton of antibodies and over time a small amount of that antibody would get in and change the equilibrium."

To most scientists, the idea would immediately have seemed like a nonstarter because of the famous blood-brain barrier, the protective mechanism that keeps carbohydrates, proteins, metals, and other impurities out of the brain. While the rest of the body's organs can easily tolerate a rich and coarse blood flow, the brain's fine vasculature cannot. Brain arteries are a delicate silk web as compared to the body's rope artery hammock, and would easily clog and burst under the pressure of such bulky particles.

The brain does need fresh blood, though, which delivers a constant infusion of oxygen and glucose in order for it to survive. So it relies on a fine mesh filter system—the blood-brain barrier. Schenk was very familiar with the barrier through some recent research he had done—so familiar that he was mindful of something that most other neuroscientists seemed not to be: The blood-brain barrier *is not perfect.* For whatever reason, it has a tiny built-in leak—about three out of every thousand unwanted particles get in.

Schenk's epiphany was that a body constantly manufacturing its own supply of beta-amyloid antibody would produce so much of it that three parts per thousand would be plenty.

Like so many other breakthroughs in history, his eureka moment capped off years of hard work. Schenk and his colleagues had been researching Alzheimer's aggressively on several fronts since 1987. With no expectation of near-term profit, they'd invested tens of millions of dollars. "For years, we've had a major, major, major commitment to Alzheimer's research, far more than any single university center," Schenk boasted. "It has been a giant effort. At one point, we had sixty people working on it at once, and that doesn't count the labs of our collaborators. It's not by chance that we came up with the vaccine. It really isn't chance."

For the vaccine experiment, Schenk cordoned off three groups of mice genetically designed to develop plaque-filled brains. The first batch, the control group, received no vaccine. The second group received a series of injections of vaccine beginning at six weeks of age (young adulthood). The third group started getting injections at twelve months (old age)—only after they had started to accumulate plaques.

After about a year, mice from groups one and two were sacrificed and dissected: Brains from the control group were, as expected, riddled with plaques. Of the nine mice in the group receiving the vaccine from early on, though, seven had virtually no plaques; the remaining two had significantly fewer than the control mice. The results were so dramatic, Schenk says, that when they first looked at the tissue slides, "we thought maybe the animals had been mixed up."

They had not. To an extent beyond the Elan team's wildest expectations, the injected bits of beta-amyloid had evidently stimulated the immune system to attack and dissolve the plaque deposits as they were being formed. It is a two-step process. First, the injected beta-amyloid prompted the immune system to tag all beta-amyloid in the brain for removal. Then white blood cells and another class of cells called microglia, acting as the body's garbage collectors, swept through and picked up everything that had been tagged. The result: no more plaques. Individual strands of beta-amyloid floating free were nabbed before they could glom on to a plaque.

Eighteen months after the experiment began, they got even better news. When they sacrificed the third group of mice—those who received the vaccine only as elderly mice—they again saw fewer plaques compared to the control group at that same age. The vaccine not only prevented plaques from forming, but also disassembled and removed plaques already in the brain. It was a true plaque-buster—not just a shield but also an antidote.

This new drug, temporarily named AN 1792, was not by any means a certain cure for Alzheimer's disease. First, the company would have to see if it was safe in humans. There was a serious worry among some neuroscientists that the injected beta-amyloid could stimulate a troublesome (possibly even lethal) autoimmune response, wherein the immune system behaves as though the body's own cells are a foreign enemy needing to be destroyed. (Other autoimmune disorders include psoriasis, rheumatoid arthritis, lupus, diabetes mellitus, and multiple sclerosis.)

Another possible scenario was that the vaccine could prove safe but ineffective. It might not clear away human plaques as effectively as mouse plaques.

Finally, of course, the vaccine might work brilliantly but not end the disease. No one could say for sure that clearing away the plaques would be enough to beat Alzheimer's.

These were serious hurdles, but all the same, Elan's announcement seemed to have inaugurated a new era in Alzheimer's research: *the beginning of the end.* This particular drug might not be the cure, but at least it was the first contender.

Yesterday when I visited my mother at the new home, she had taken her outer garments off and was taking a nap in someone else's bed (alone). Her personal teddy bear was in someone else's room. This is one of her best friends, and she used to constantly carry it around and talk to it. I rescued it and put it in her arms as she slept. I realize that residents take things from others' rooms, but feel bad that her teddy bear was not close by her.

The old house had five to eight residents. This new one has sixteen. She has sixteen closets to hide in. The staff is cautious when opening closets, because Mother will jump out and "boo" them.

—J.T.
Cross Plains, Wisconsin

Chapter 15

ONE THOUSAND SUBTRACTIONS

·◌·

The late years of Ralph Waldo Emerson's senile dementia were probably about as peaceful as anyone could have hoped. "He suffered very little," wrote his son Edward, "took his nourishment well, but had great annoyance from his inability to find the words which he wished for. . . . He went to his study and tried to work, accomplished less and less, but did not notice it." Emerson became intermittently confused about where he was, lost his ability to write letters and to understand what he was reading and much of what was said to him, and lost grasp entirely of many important figures in his life. Within a week of Henry Wadsworth Longfellow's death, in the spring of 1882, Emerson could not be made to understand *who* his old friend was. The entity of "Longfellow" in Emerson's mind had comprised a broad constellation of synapses, and that particular constellation was now inaccessible. Did it still exist? Only as cellular residue.

By far the most vivid account of Emerson's late-stage dementia comes to us via the efforts of an industrious and conniving young man named Edward Bok. A Dutch immigrant who settled in New York City with his family in 1870, when he was seven, Bok quickly became smitten by the unrelenting American can-do spirit, and particularly seduced by the allure of celebrity. By his early teens, as an office boy at Western Union Telegraph and a budding freelance reporter, he developed an ambition to meet and interact (however superficially) with the most popular public figures of the time. Emerson was near the top of Bok's wish list.

After easily engaging former President Ulysses S. Grant and then-President Rutherford B. Hayes, Bok traveled to Boston to make more famous "friends" and collect their autographs. Just eighteen, he was already savvy enough to understand how one association could lead to another, and planned his visits accordingly. Over the course of just a few days in November 1881, Bok parlayed a meeting with Oliver Wendell Holmes into one with Longfellow; the Longfellow interaction begat an audience with the Episcopal bishop Phillips Brooks (composer of "O Little Town of Bethlehem"). Brooks, in turn, advised Bok on how to see Emerson. "I don't know whether you will see him at his *best,*" he warned the young man in polite understatement. Bok had no idea what he was talking about.

The next day Bok went to Concord, where he managed to enchant *Little Women* author Louisa May Alcott. Now nearly fifty, Alcott had grown up with Emerson as a neighbor and uncle figure. "Our best and greatest American," she called him in her journal, ". . . and the man who has helped me most by his life, his books, his society." Alcott agreed to make an introduction for Bok, while also warning him that Emerson was not the man he once had been.

When they arrived at the house, though, Ellen Emerson politely declined to show them in. "Father sees no one now," she said, "and I fear it might not be a pleasure if you did see him." Bok was prepared for this contingency. At just the right moment, he expertly dropped in a line from his previous day's conversation with Phillips Brooks, and once again a door opened.

The vacant ghost of Emerson was sitting quietly at the desk in his study. "Father," said Ellen, gently alerting Emerson to his uninvited guests. He looked up at them and smiled, but said nothing. Then, slowly rising from his desk, he offered his hand and gestured vaguely toward some empty chairs. But as soon as he had turned away for just a moment, something very unsettling happened: Emerson wandered away from his visitors and toward the window. There, he stood for a while, apparently oblivious to any other presence in the room. In a split instant, he seemed to have forgotten entirely about the others.

Ellen, who had been slowly losing her father for more than a dozen years, started to cry and left the room, but Louisa and Edward stayed on quietly. After a few minutes, Emerson headed back to his desk, noticing them along the way. Again, he bowed a silent greeting, then sat down at the desk; once more, out of sight, out of mind.

What no doctor in 1881 could have known was that Emerson was by now operating with a virtually obliterated hippocampus, occasioning a virtually perfect case of anterograde amnesia—the loss of ability to create any new memories. If his was an Alzheimer's pathology, plaques and tangles germinating in the hippocampal formation had first started to create a noticeable disturbance in Emerson's functioning almost fifteen years earlier. Since that time, as the unwelcome particles spread to other regions of the brain, they also continued to proliferate in their original nest. Slowly, steadily, a critical mass of neurons and connections between neurons had been hacked apart; probably no more than half of the original healthy cells now remained. In this state, not only was the hippocampus completely incapable of consolidating short-term into long-term memories; it could not even establish "working memories" of a duration of minutes.

All that was left, then, was a limited capacity for "immediate memory" of mere seconds. Emerson was still conscious, and somewhat sentient. He could still coalesce different fields of information—verbal, visual, auditory—into a cogent sense of the present tense, a working (if constricted) consciousness. He was still, in some sense, *there*.

But how much of the great mind remained was an open question. Gently probing that consciousness for its eroding boundary, his old friend Louisa now spoke up in a nervous attempt to end the dreadful silence in the room.

"Have you read this new book by Ruskin yet?" she asked.

The voice didn't register. Emerson rose slowly and looked up at Louisa. "Did you speak to me, madam?" he asked. At the moment, he had no apparent recognition of a friend of nearly half a century—the realization of which sent Louisa into tears. As she retreated to the other side of the room, Bok, now left alone with Emerson, saw his opportunity and blurted out his long-planned request.

"I thought, perhaps, Mr. Emerson, that you might be able to favor me with a letter from Carlyle."

"Carlyle? Did you say Carlyle?"

"Yes," repeated Bok. "Thomas Carlyle."

"Yes, to be sure. Carlyle. Yes, he was here this morning. He will be here again tomorrow morning." In fact, as even Bok knew, Carlyle lived in England. The two had not seen each other for many years.

There was a pause, into which Emerson lost his train of thought. Emerson looked at the boy for a cue. "You were saying?"

Bok repeated his request. Could Emerson give him one of the original Carlyle letters?

"Oh, I think so, I think so. Let me see. Yes, here in this drawer I have many letters from Carlyle." He ruffled through some papers in his desk drawer and then again lost himself. More quiet moments passed. Finally, Bok, sensing correctly that his visit was about to come to an end, pared down his request. He asked for a simple autograph.

"Mr. Emerson," Bok said, "will you be so good as to write your name in this book for me?"

"Name?" said a puzzled Emerson.

"Yes, please. Your name: Ralph Waldo Emerson."

"Please write out the name you want, and I will copy it for you if I can."

Bok, stunned, wrote out "Ralph Waldo Emerson, Concord, November 22, 1881," on a slip of paper and handed it to Emerson along with the book. Emerson then copied Bok's dictation, very slowly copying letter by letter:

R. Waldo Emerson
Conocord
November 22, 1881

(Notice the extra "o" in Concord. In his fog, Emerson had misspelled the town which he himself had made world-famous.)

After the autograph came the most chilling occurrence yet. Emerson forgot about signing his name just as soon as he had done so. A few moments after Bok placed the autograph book back in his pocket, Emerson caught sight of the slip with Bok's handwriting on his desk and fell into a wide smile.

"You wish me to write my name?" he said. "With pleasure. Have you a book with you?"

Bok, now "overcome with astonishment," again handed him the autograph book. And so it was that Emerson autographed Bok's book not once but twice, bestowing on the young man two separate handwritten pieces of evidence of having met the great Transcendentalist in person—when, as a matter of both neurobiology and humanity, he had arguably never met Emerson at all.

Two weeks later, Emerson was dead, of pneumonia.

If Emerson was, as it appears in medical hindsight, afflicted with a reasonably straightforward case of what we now call Alzheimer's disease, it is also clear that he was mercifully released from the scripted drama before its dismal finale. In the end, for those Alzheimer's sufferers who do not die of something else along the way—pneumonia, stroke, heart failure, cancer, etc.—speech dissolves completely, incontinence sets in, muscles become stiff, walking becomes impossible; the face loses all elasticity, breathing becomes labored, swallowing ceases. All of this happens slowly, incrementally, insidiously, over months or even years.

In the brain, the pathway of the disease is the steady continuation of retrogenesis completing its relentless undoing on the way back to birth, the plaques and tangles moving into those regions that control gross motor function and are the very first to become myelinated in an infant.

Stage

7c	Can no longer walk without assistance
7d	Can no longer sit up without assistance
7e	Can no longer smile
7f	Can no longer hold up head

After the motor skills begin to collapse, limiting the patient to a wheelchair and then to a bed; after the eyes lose their ability to focus, something happens that is chilling even for this disease: the return of the infant reflexes.

In normal development, infants younger than six months will, when the soles of their feet are stimulated, raise their big toe up and spread their other toes outward. This is called the Babinski sign, after the French neurologist Joseph François Félix Babinski, who first described the phenomenon in 1903. The Babinski sign disappears after approximately six months of age; from then on the toes reflex downward in response to the same stimulus. Alzheimer's patients reclaim the Babinski sign (also now called the plantar response) in the very late stages, along with the other well-known infant reflexes: rooting, sucking, grasping. They all come back. If you scratch the palm of a late-stage patient, you might notice a twitch of the chin muscle on the same side. If you put your finger in the palm of his hand, you'll feel an instant, familiar grab.

After much of the cortex has been decimated, and thinking and mobility are all but at an end, the tangles launch their final assault on the brain in its most primitive and evolutionarily oldest region: the brainstem, at the base of the brain, just above the spinal cord. The brainstem controls involuntary, hard-wired functions such as breathing, blinking, blood pressure, heart rate, and sleeping cycles. It regulates the lungs, intestines, liver, kidneys, pancreas, and other organs, freeing up the cortex to worry about sensations, movements, and ideas. A person with extensive cortical damage but an intact brainstem can live for years in a "persistent vegetative state" with feeding tubes and meticulous care. But Alzheimer's does not let that happen. It finishes the job by slowly destroying the brainstem just as it has destroyed the hippocampus and the other regions of the brain along the way.

No matter how long the end has been anticipated by friends and family, no one knows quite what to expect. On the Alzheimer List, Stephanie Zeman, a nurse specializing in dementia care, counseled her listmates about the final path toward death. "The last few days of life for most people with dementia," she said, "go something like this: The person will stop taking anything by mouth. They may sleep a lot. At this point families worry about the discomfort of hunger or thirst. Studies indicate that at this stage the person does not experience discomfort from either hunger or thirst because the body is literally shutting down. This is a natural process. The digestive system and kidneys can no longer process nutrients or eliminate waste normally. Loading the system with IV fluids often puts the person into congestive heart failure and their lungs may become congested because the heart is also beginning to fail and cannot pump the larger blood volume any more.

"The hands and feet will begin to feel cold and may develop what is called mottling, a blotchy look, because now some of the tissues are not getting a normal level of oxygen. The person is now fairly unresponsive and their breathing becomes shallower and may sound noisy from an accumulation of fluids in their throat. At this point the head can be elevated slightly and turned to the side to help with this. This stage may last a day or more. Hands and feet are now very cold. Family may want to put blankets on the person but in fact, as the body shuts down, it conserves all of its resources for the trunk and brain so the core body temperature is not sub-normal but may in fact, be elevated. A light sheet is usually all that is needed.

"The end of life is usually very quiet and the person just slips away. Families at the bedside may suddenly realize the person is not breathing any more. Within a few minutes the heart stops and the person is truly at rest."

Life passes, and the caregiver can no longer give care. Into the void rushes a powerful sea of emotion, with uneven waves of relief, regret, guilt, anger, emptiness, and renewed purpose. On the surface, the caregiver is finally cut loose from an extraordinary burden, and is relieved. The long decline is over.

Under any circumstances, mourning a lost life is a complex emotional event. With Alzheimer's, though, it is particularly torturous because in this long disease there have already been so many expirations along the way. In *Man's Search for Meaning*, Viktor Frankl raised the specter of "emotional death," the death of the spirit occurring well before the death of the actual body. Alzheimer's specializes in such split-level death. The final passing from Alzheimer's is really just the last in a long series of deaths. It is death not by a thousand cuts but by a thousand subtractions.

This understanding of Alzheimer's death, in turn, suggests

something important about death in general that ordinarily goes unnoticed. The truth is that, no matter the cause, death is *never* a single end but a collection of ends that are ordinarily so tightly bound together that they appear to be one entity. In the same way that visible light usually appears to be a single colorless article, death usually looks like a single experience. One moment the person is there, alive, and the next moment—*flick*—the light switches off and the person is gone. Here, then not here. The doctor looks over at the clock on the wall and quietly says, "Time of death, 11:19."

But the reality of death is not so crisp. Even when the dying is instantaneous, as from a catastrophic collision, death is not just the squelching of the heart, not just the end of oxygen to the brain, not just the cessation of energy in the body. It is the smothering of a veritable universe of living fibers, the death of billions of individual cells and trillions of connections among those cells. A constellation of memories is dissolved, as are habits, feelings, cravings, annoyances. Not just a body, but its constituent parts: ten long fingers and ten knobby toes, a playful mouth, eyes that can be piercing or despondent.

Why are so many people fascinated by Alzheimer's disease? Because it is not only a disease, but also a prism through which we can view life in ways not normally available to us. Through the Alzheimer's prism, we can experience life's constituent parts and understand better its resonances and quirks. And as the disease relentlessly progresses toward the final dimming of the sufferer, it forces us to experience death in a way it is rarely otherwise experienced. What is usually a quick flicker we see in super slow motion, over years. It is more painful than many people can even imagine, but it is also perhaps the most poignant of all reminders of why and how human life is so extraordinary. It is our best lens on the meaning of loss.

Like Emerson, Jonathan Swift did not live long enough with his progressive dementia to unravel completely. He did, though, die quite a few deaths along the way to his final passing. His late stages were marked by intensive walking, sometimes up to ten hours a day. He gradually lost access to nearly all his words and would rarely speak. Once, near the end, a servant picked up Swift's watch to find out the time. Curious, Swift managed to utter "Bring it here" and stared at the watch for some time. He also once reached for a knife; when it was taken away, he shrugged his shoulders and said, "I am what I am. I am what I am."

His last recorded words were spoken to his servant. He couldn't find the words that he wanted, and finally settled for "I am a fool." Swift died mourning the death of his own intellect. He died grieving for himself.

I had a dream three nights after Dad died: The telephone rang and I answered. Turning around I saw my father—no longer emaciated and ill with cancer, but round, rosy, and healthy. He put his arms around me and said, "I just want you to know that everything's all right."

Strange, but I had no such dream about Mother returning after her death. Alzheimer's had taken so much from her and from us that she, literally, didn't seem to linger here on earth. As my daughter said, "It's almost like Grandma said, 'I'm outta here!'" Who can blame her?

However, shortly after her death my father returned in a dream, wearing an absolutely terrible red plaid jacket. (Only mother could have gotten him to wear that thing! She loved red plaid.) He said that Mother had sent him to tell me they were together and all was well.

I learned to not be afraid to hurt. I learned to get all the help I needed in order to heal. As a result I'm beginning to remember the happier side of Mother.

—S.P.
Denver, Colorado

Chapter 16

THINGS TO AVOID

᠙

Doctors cannot yet cure Alzheimer's, or prevent it, or even mask its symptoms for very long. But hundreds of studies have begun to produce a pointillist portrait of how people can help themselves— things to do for the body, mind, and spirit that *might* reduce the risk of getting the disease, or at least delay its onset:

Avoid head injuries.

Avoid fatty foods.

Avoid high blood pressure.

Eat foods rich in antioxidants, which eliminate damaging free-radical molecules. Eat, specifically: prunes, raisins, blueberries, blackberries, kale, strawberries, spinach, raspberries, brussels sprouts, plums, alfalfa sprouts, broccoli, beets, oranges, red grapes, red peppers, and cherries. (Foods listed according to their antioxidant content, in descending order.)

Eat foods rich in folic acid, and in vitamins B6, B12, C, and E.

Eat tuna, salmon, and other foods rich in fatty acids.

Don't drink too much alcohol. (A moderate amount might be slightly beneficial.)

Don't skimp on sleep. (Sleep is rejuvenating to the brain and the body; sleep seems to play a very important role in long-term memory formation.)

Exercise.

Maintain a high level of social contact (and consider marriage—one study shows fewer married people getting Alzheimer's).

If you are a woman past menopause, consider estrogen replacement therapy. (Some studies suggest it may reduce Alzheimer's incidence by as much as half.)

If you like to chew gum, continue chewing gum. (This is very tentative. One study suggests a mysterious connection between chewing and the health of hippocampal cells.)

If you regularly take nonsteroidal anti-inflammatory drugs such as ibuprofen for another reason, continue. (Some studies show a benefit.)

Get a thorough education.

Keep your mind active. Read, discuss, debate, create, play word games, do crossword puzzles, meet new people, learn new languages. Studies show that people with very high levels of education, while not immune from Alzheimer's, do tend to get the disease later than others.

Ancients in Greece and Rome did not have to be goaded into keeping their minds limber. They had no choice. By necessity, they relied on mind and memory to an extent that people today would find hard to believe. The men that Emerson admired in his journal—"L. Scipio knew the name of every man in Rome. . . . Seneca could say two thousand words in one hearing"—had no convenient alternative. There was no printing press, no pen and ink; the cumbersome wax tablet was the best external device they had. So the mind was always the default notebook of choice.

To put it to the most efficient use possible, the Greeks invented *mnemonics*—a technique to assist memory. The art of mnemonics (pronounced *neh-MON-iks)* was built around the observation that while the human capacity to remember ideas, language, and numbers seems frightfully limited, visual memory is nearly infallible. The hackneyed phrase "I never forget a face" turns out to be a literal fact of human biology; in tests running into the thousands of faces, there seems to be no limit to powers of recognition. By contrast, remembering a string of fifteen to twenty numbers is a strenuous chore.

The strange disparity between visual memory and word/number memory impressed Greek intellectuals somewhere around the fourth century B.C. The legend is that mnemonics was first demonstrated by the poet Simonides of Ceos (556–468 B.C.), the sole survivor in the collapse of a large banquet hall. Simonides had just stepped outside the hall to receive a message when the roof caved in and crushed everyone inside. To his surprise, the poet found that he was able to reel off a flawless list of the victims, and to identify each crushed body. He did this by recalling where each person had been sitting in the banquet hall. It was as if he had a tiny map of the banquet hall imprinted somewhere in his brain.

We all do. Neuroscientists would later discover that a particular region of the hippocampus is filled with "place cells" programmed to create cellular landscape maps from visual perception. While not photographically flawless in their registration of detail, these place cells help us recall the position of an object in relation to the position of other objects. Recall that in the very early stages of Ronald Reagan's illness, he turned to his wife and said, "Well, I've got to wait a minute. I'm not quite sure where I am." The early destruction of hippocampal place cells in Alzheimer's disease is the reason for sudden "Where-am-I?" moments. Much like a brittle old road map in the closet, the spatial map in Reagan's brain was disintegrating.

With only an intuitive understanding of place cells, the Greeks went on to develop a series of mnemonic devices rooted in the power of visual memory. Many were based on the architectural model that Simonides had inspired—a visualization of rooms in a home, for example, into which the mnemonist would "deposit" pieces of information: one name on a dining room table, another name in the fireplace, yet another in the hallway, and so on. Over time, people found that, with the right devices, the brain could be turned into a startlingly reliable reference tool.

Mnemonics proved to be a critical tool in the long human struggle toward enlightenment. So-called memory palaces and memory theaters were a dominant feature of the intellectual landscape for more than a thousand years, well through the Renaissance. The historian Frances Yates suggests that Shakespeare's Globe Theater was actually based on the model of a memory theater. "I come to the fields and vast palaces of memory," Saint Augustine wrote in *Confessions*. "Hidden there is whatever . . . has been deposited and placed on reserve and has not been swallowed up and buried in oblivion. When I am in this storehouse, I ask that it produce what

I want to recall, and immediately certain things come out; some things require a longer search, and have to be drawn out as it were from more recondite receptacles."

Today, we treat the brain differently. Even those who think for a living don't rely on it as a data storehouse. In place of the vast internal memory palace, we have Post-it Notes, steno notebooks, Palm Pilots, libraries, and the Internet. We are awash in external memory, upon which we have built edifying worlds of art, literature, science, law, and philosophy. The modern brain is saved primarily for synthesis of ideas, emotional impressions, rhetorical flair, and amusement.

In the transformation, we have surrendered some of memory's importance. In 2001, I do not need to remember a long list of names (I write them down), or the full text of a speech (I use note cards or a TelePrompTer), or every bone and blood vessel in the body (I can refer to a textbook). I do not need to know how to calculate a circumference (calculator), or even how to spell "calculator" (spell checker). I just need to know that these information resources exist, and how to use them. This is one of the essential truths of the post-Gutenberg age: We live in a world of shared information and understanding—the challenge is not to know it all, but to know how to know. "Our age is retrospective," Emerson wrote in *Nature.* "It builds the sepulchres of the fathers. It writes biographies, histories, and criticism. The foregoing generations beheld God and nature face-to-face; we, through their eyes."

Shared understanding and memory is an obvious step forward in human civilization, but it is not without its trade-offs. Emerson's chief worry was that the flood of knowledge from others would cut us off from the wisdom of personal experience. But he was also very concerned by the steady loss of life-affirming skills due to the gradual adoption of more and more labor-saving and thought-saving conveniences. "The civilized man has built a coach," he said, "but has lost the use of his feet. He is supported on crutches, but lacks so much support of muscle. He has a fine Geneva watch, but he fails of the skill to tell the hour by the sun. . . . His notebooks impair his memory; his libraries overload his wit . . . and it may be a question whether machinery does not encumber; whether we have not lost by refinement some energy . . . some vigor of wild virtue."

It was not a new warning, even then. Plato had cautioned two thousand years before that the new tool of writing was "a recipe not for memory, but for reminder." He prophesied a world with more external knowledge and less internal proficiency: "If men learn this, it will implant forgetfulness in their souls: they will cease to exercise memory because they rely on that which is written."

The lesser-used mind does, almost inevitably, become a somewhat weaker instrument. Is it possible, in our superior modern world, with terabytes of instantly accessible knowledge and machines that practically think for us, that even healthy brains are in something of an insidious decline? We know that labor-saving devices like cars and washing machines have led to couch-potato lifestyles and a steady rise in obesity. What we don't recognize quite so readily is a corresponding link between the rise of external memory and a decrease in brain exertion. Not doing the mental work means not building those internal connections between neurons.

We use our brains to build great tools that make our lives safer, cleaner, longer, easier. But these same tools also dull our minds.

Not surprisingly, modern science has already risen to treat this emerging problem. The start of the twenty-first century saw neuroscientists classifying mild memory loss as a new disease: mild cognitive impairment (MCI). Society seems eager for this, already flocking to herbal tonics like adrafinil, deprenyl, gingko biloba, and piracetam as potential medical solutions to cognitive frustration.

It is intrinsically human to want to better ourselves with tools. But there may also be a price paid in the quest. Of all the quantitative perks acquired through technological progress—convenience, efficiency, longevity, the thrill of electronic contact—none add a whit to the one true qualitative pursuit: to make life more meaningful. To the contrary, the manic chase of material improvements can easily crowd out the pursuit of meaning.

If material gains are spiritually empty, the obverse is also true: hardship or loss can offer a window to spiritual transcendence. "The helpless victim of a hopeless situation," Viktor Frankl says, "facing a fate he cannot change, may rise above himself, may grow beyond himself, and by so doing, change himself."

Finding meaning through loss: it is an observation that anyone who has flunked a test, skinned a knee, or lost a friend can easily relate to. Meaning through loss is one of life's chief—and most reliable and universal—paradoxes.

While it is perfectly understandable, then, to want to *overcome* loss—and we all yearn to, and always will—it's equally important to remember loss's utility. If Alzheimer's is, as I have already argued, one of our best lenses on life and the meaning of loss, then the medical war on Alzheimer's presents two substantial dangers:

1. We may get so distracted by the goal of defeating Alzheimer's that we lose sight of the disease's essential humanity.

2. In winning the war, should we be so fortunate, we will also be eliminating the lens that has served humanity so well for thousands of years. Defeating Alzheimer's will be like defeating winter. Once it is gone, we'll face less hardship, but we'll also have lost one of life's reliable touchstones.

The same lesson applies to other scientific ambitions. Since we now have the power to overcome nature—to tinker with our own genetics—it is crucial to try to realize what we'll be giving up as we overcome our limitations. The burden ultimately rests with non-scientists to insist on a full exploration of these issues, since very few scientists will stop to explore them on their own accord.

One scientific movement that presses ahead without a full consideration of the ramifications is called *posthumanism.* "We are at the point of remaking human biology," Gregory Stock, director of the Science, Technology and Society program at UCLA, wrote in 1998. Stock, author of *Metaman: The Merging of Humans and Machines into a Global Superorganism,* was talking about the virtues of germline engineering—the creation of *knock-out people* by adding and subtracting traits as we see fit. Posthumanists ask: What qualities in particular would you like your next child to have? They want to take the design process away from natural selection and put it in the hands of individual human beings.

Now that we have transgenic mice with muscular dystrophy and asthma, it is no great stretch of the imagination to think about scientists manipulating human genes to enhance the prowess of the brain. Is the power of memory a gene-based trait? The man with the perfect memory, A. R. Luria's remarkable human subject S., would have said so. Both his parents also had otherworldly memories, as did a cousin. In 1995, Tim Tully, a scientist at Cold Spring Harbor on Long Island, kicked off the brain-enhancement era with an insect counterpart to S., a transgenic fly that forms scent memories much faster than ordinary flies and keeps them forever. He called it the fly with photographic memory.

Advocates of germline engineering imagine a world not too far away that will be populated by "posthumans." Our post-human children, they predict, will have faster, more reliable brains, germ-resistant bodies, and other adaptations that make us clearly better. The apotheosis of posthumanism is the death of death: the "manufacturing" of an unlimited amount of time for humans to enjoy life. "I am now working on immortality," University of California at Irvine evolutionary biologist Michael Rose told *Wired* magazine for its January 2000 issue. Rose is not the only serious scientist aiming to obliterate life's ultimate boundary. The Silicon Valley genetic engineering firm Geron is trying to unlock the secrets of telomerase, an enzyme found in sperm cells and cancer cells that seems to be the key to keeping such cells youthful. Another corporate stem-cell researcher, William Haseltine, founder of Human Genome Sciences, predicted that this research arc will lead to what he called a "transubstantiated future" for human beings within seventy years—meaning that the generation born in the late twentieth century could be the last to face death as an inevitability.

The number of obstacles to immortality make it impossible to guess seriously about whether it will ever happen. But its plausibility demands that we begin to ask: *Do we want this?* Do we want perfect memories and endless lives?

In *Gulliver's Travels,* Gulliver changes his mind about the glories of immortality after he sees that it is fraught with problems. But what about a *clean* immortality, one that would actually work well? What if, short of eternity, we could live four hundred relatively healthy years instead of seventy-five? Imagine being able to stick around and see your children's children's children's children's children's children's children's children's children's children's children's children's children's children's children's children. If we could do so in sound mind and relatively sound body, without being too much of a burden on our families or our communities, we could indeed live out the original aspirations of Gulliver—to first acquire great material wealth and a formidable education and then spend subsequent lifetimes putting those resources to great use, pursuing modernization, universal health care, and other high-minded humanistic pursuits.

It sounds wonderful, and perhaps would be in many ways. But it would also be a fundamental challenge to how we understand ourselves, and it is almost impossible to imagine the ramifications—good and bad—for humanity.

To be human as we know it today is to experience the cycles of life, to experience great loss and pain—not just the pain of tragedy but the pain of inevitability. The essential joy of life is embedded in our mortality, and in our forgetting. How we would be changing ourselves if we decide to cross the Rubicon to posthumanity is impossible to tell. Life as we know it is an incalculably complicated web of interdependence. Species rely on other species for survival, and abilities and capacities are balanced out by other abilities or inabilities. But more important than the unintended consequences of manipulating DNA is the essential loss of humanity that happens as soon as we begin doing so. As Plato, Nietzsche, Emerson, and others have argued, humanity is something we should savor for all of its frailties as well as its abilities. The only true wisdom, said Joseph Campbell in a paraphrase of the Caribou Eskimo Shaman Igjugarjuk, "lives far from mankind, out in the great loneliness, and can be reached only through suffering. Privation and suffering alone open the mind to all that is hidden to others."

One cannot appreciate life's majesty without experiencing its hardships. In the Wim Wenders film *Wings of Desire,* angels abandon a perfect but colorless heaven for a life on earth with all of its Technicolor problems. Perfection is boring and lifeless; reality, with its grit and loss, is fulfilling.

Perhaps no human being has experienced this hard truth as completely as S., the man with the perfect memory. Recall that although he remembered everything he ever came into contact with, S. could make sense of almost nothing. Simple stories baffled him, and even people's faces were difficult for him to place because he recorded so much information about each moment's expression. S. spent his entire life looking at everything with a magnifying glass, taking in so many details that he could never pull back far enough to make sense of the patterns. He saw the trees but not the forest. "The big question for him, and the most troublesome," wrote Luria, "was how he could learn to forget. . . . there were numerous details in the text, each of which gave rise to new images that led him far afield, until his mind was a virtual chaos. How could he avoid these images, prevent himself from seeing details which kept him from understanding a simple story? . . . The problem of forgetting . . . became a torment for him."

S. tried everything he could think of to forget. He tried writing things down, reasoning that if he wrote something down he wouldn't need to remember it, would be free to forget it. "But I got nowhere," he reported. "For in my mind, I continued to see what I'd written." Even when he tried writing everything down on the same sort of paper with the same pencil, the information would not blur together as he'd hoped. He kept seeing it all distinctly in his mind's eye.

So he tried burning it, literally. He would record information on paper, set it afire and then watch the paper burn into a charred scrap. But that didn't work either. In his mind, he still saw the information under the black char.

The image of a man literally burning information in his struggle to forget is perhaps the most poignant way to marvel at memory and its gorgeous fragility. Our limitations *are* our strengths. Perhaps it is true that with very slight modifications our brains and bodies could be made virtually invulnerable. But in escaping loss we would also be escaping life.

We are like the dead in Thornton Wilder's Our Town. *As we drift away from life, no longer fearing to die nor craving and striving for our place in the sun, we can look back on the world that was, and see it as a whole.*

—Morris Friedell

Chapter 17

THE MICE ARE SMARTER

~.~

Washington Hilton, Washington, D.C.: July 2000

Near the entrance to this hotel nineteen years ago, John Hinckley crouched to his knees and opened fire on Ronald Reagan and his staff, as the President left the building following a speech to labor union delegates.

Now Reagan's daughter Maureen returned to this place of dreadful memory to address another assembly, the World Alzheimer Congress. It was the largest-ever professional gathering on the disease.

Her father was in the final stages. He had stopped talking, and was having some trouble walking. Maureen, meanwhile, had emerged as a powerful voice in the crusade against Alzheimer's, skillfully using her family's public tragedy to raise awareness and to campaign for more government research funding. In the Hilton's expansive basement conference center, she joined physicians, nurses, counselors, and more than three thousand researchers for a broad review of the latest scientific developments and caregiving techniques.

There was also a pack of journalists. Everyone wanted to hear the bulletin about Dale Schenk's vaccine—about how the knock-out mice were getting *smarter.*

The vaccine really seemed to be working, at least in animals. A number of labs around the world had replicated Schenk's results, and one had gone further. At the University of South Florida, re-searchers gave vaccine injections to the knock-out mice and then months later tested their memories. They found just what they'd hoped: In water mazes, the mice did not bumble about the way they had been genetically designed to; instead, they learned how to navigate the maze just like normal mice. They were normal now, apparently. For these humanized mice, at least, Alzheimer's disease was now preventable.

This has to be taken in context, of course: Mice don't really get Alzheimer's, so they can't really be cured of it. The mice whose brains had been artificially contaminated with plaques had now been artificially cleansed of them; it *seemed* like a step in the right direction, but one had to remember that a disease that only exists in humans can only be cured in humans.

In a small room crowded with microphones and cables, Schenk and his boss Ivan Lieberburg gave a briefing to an interna-tional press corps, sharing even better news: Phase I safety trials had ended with no observable side effects of the vaccine on hu-mans. Phase II multidose human trials would therefore soon com-mence, this time to test the drug's effectiveness. They could have the first results in as few as eighteen months—at the end of 2001. That's when the world would first get an inkling of whether or not this was going to be a useful treatment for Alzheimer's, or a cure, or nothing at all.

That same morning, Schenk shared the fine points with fellow researchers in the hotel's underground ballroom. Reviewing the data from follow-up studies on mice, guinea pigs, rabbits, and monkeys, he said it was now clear that the vaccine was working exactly as they predicted: The injected beta-amyloid was prompting the immune systems to produce targeted antibodies, a small portion of which were crossing the blood-brain barrier and binding directly with beta-amyloid in the brain. Then the offending substances were effortlessly being cleared away as cellular trash.

Even though most of these scientists had known something about the vaccine for almost a year, many still seemed startled to hear Schenk's presentation. Just a few years earlier, no one could have even imagined that anyone would be talking about a potential cure so soon. It was as if President Kennedy had called for a moon landing within a decade and NASA soon reported back that they were about to land men on Mars.

After the talk, as everyone filed out of the large ballroom to head for the smaller specialized sessions of the day, one researcher turned to another and asked, "So if this thing works, is the game over?"

On the surface, of course, that was the big question: Will clearing the plaques abolish this disease? Going deeper, though, there was a more fundamental question raised by this vaccine's sudden emergence: Why had Dale Schenk been the only person on earth to think of it? And why had he been laughed out of the room when he first shared his thought?

It was a variation on the recurring theme of outcast scientists. Why was Stanley Prusiner vilified for years over his unusual—but as it turned out, correct—idea about infectious prions? Why was Allen Roses denied grants for follow-up research to his important ApoE discovery? Why was Ruth Itzhaki ignored in her pursuit of herpes simplex virus 1? Why was Meta Neumann ignored? Alois Alzheimer? Why does the culture of science seem to so often punish the most inventive?

Science is ultimately a human endeavor. Its language is uniform, its methods are strict, but the questions posed and the analysis applied are as idiosyncratic as love affairs and operas and football games. There is, thus, an organic incongruity. Scientific discovery is, and always will be, an inherently clumsy matter as scientists attempt to fit the round peg of humanity into the square hole of objectivity.

The most adventuresome of these scientists, pushing against the limits of comprehension, are inevitably bruised by the friction. They are threatening existing power structures and, perhaps more dangerously, jeopardizing people's basic understanding of the world around them. They are casting doubt on "truths" on top of which people have built their careers, and around which they have oriented their lives. If a scientist named Galileo suggests in the early seventeenth century that the earth revolves around the sun, the veracity of that statement does not matter nearly as much to his peers as how its consideration may immediately affect their lives. So Galileo is forced to recant. That particular truth will have to wait.

The persistent challenge of science, and all edification, is to minimize the friction: to encourage the pursuit of new ideas while helping to sustain the integrity of people's lives.

Other enticing developments were revealed at the July 2000 conference. Researchers from the Mayo Clinic had just produced the first knock-out mouse with both plaques *and* tangles. Several drug companies had isolated the brain enzyme that seems to convert harmless APP into malicious beta-amyloid; perhaps a drug could arrest that process. "There's a smell of success in the air," said the NIA's Marcelle Morrison-Bogorad.

Hundreds of more mundane, if still important, presentations were also taking place. In the Jefferson Room, New York University's Yaakov Stern was comparing the hippocampal memory network with the prefrontal memory network; in the Monroe Room the University of Texas's Rachel Doody was reviewing the limited success of Aricept and other similar drugs.

The real heart of the conference, though, was in the free-for-all poster sessions at midday. In a vast, low-ceilinged room, the entire community of researchers came together every day at noon to eat bland sandwiches and browse the hundreds of large bulletin board presentations lined up in long rows. These were novel bits of research from experiments, many of which were still in progress. It was old-fashioned science, with data open for review and critique. Charts were pinned next to graphs, were pinned next to microscopic photographs, were pinned next to project summaries, were pinned next to tentative conclusions, were pinned next to contact information. Gerontologists from Sweden huddled in front of one poster, right next to a group of microbiologists from New Orleans. There was barely enough room to squeeze through.

The variety of material was fierce.

Poster #40, presented by Tohru Hasegawa, discussed the potential preventative effect of Japanese green tea.

Poster #96, presented by R. Distl & V. Meske, revealed that microdensitofluorometrically determined free cholesterol is higher in tangle-bearing neurons than in tangle-free neurons.

Poster #168, presented by Jennifer W. Catania *et al*, reviewed the genetics of Alzheimer's disease in the Caribbean Hispanic population.

The paradox of these poster sessions, and of the entire scientific portion of the conference, was that amidst all the data and ideas the *disease* was nowhere to be found. Science had fragmented it into almost unrecognizable shards—cholinergic transmitters, vascular risk factors, nicotinic receptors, aspartyl proteases, synaptic plasticity in mice, and on and on. The crowd had the patina of a large cohesive community, but was really a collection of superbly focused specialists—most of whom barely knew how to talk to anyone outside their constricted microfield. In the name of science, good science, they were far too close to the trees to see the forest.

It would take a trailblazer to try to show them the panoramic view. On the last day of the conference, in the last row of the poster session bazaar, the very final display stood out from the others. It had an entirely different flavor:

#1231

POTENTIAL FOR REHABILITATION IN ALZHEIMER'S

Standing beside #1231 was a man in a brown tweed coat and a graying beard: Morris Friedell, the college professor from Santa Barbara. Struggling to maintain his dignity and his wits as Alzheimer's slowly advanced, he had made the long journey from out west to present his ideas to the community of scientists. Until now, conversations about his ambitious ideas had mostly been limited to fellow victims, caregivers, friends, and family. His dream was to share them with professionals. He thought he might be onto something important. From his poster:

Central hypothesis:
The typical qualitative symptoms of mild to moderate Alzheimer's, gross forgetfulness, disorientation, and loss of abstraction and judgment, stem from quantitative decrements in processing capacity underlying these functions. Since patients retain substantial strength in procedural memory and memory for emotionally significant events, there is major potential for rehabilitation through relearning activities using a greater number of simpler steps.

The complex presentation contained fragments of neurobiology, sports psychology, and spirituality. There were quotes from Frankl, Thoreau, and Lao-tzu ("In the pursuit of learning, every day something is acquired. In the pursuit of Tao, every day something is dropped.") There were poems from victims, a color copy of a de Kooning from 1984, and a diagram from the psychologist A. R. Luria demonstrating rehabilitation of a brain-damaged patient. Morris's own PET scan report was also pinned up on display. Appended to the conclusion was a note: "I welcome feedback and discussion. I'm staying at———. Phone is———. E-mail is———."

But his poster drew almost no interest. Researchers peered at it for a second and moved on. They didn't know what to make of this unorthodox exhibit, and seemed anxious to find something more technical and less ambiguous—something closer to their own specialty. There was, of course, no one at this conference—or any conference—who specialized in rehabilitating Alzheimer's patients. That's just why Morris was there.

He gently looked around at the sea of researchers passing him by. "I feel like I'm living a dual life right now," he said quietly. "On the one hand, I feel like a kid at a science fair. But I also feel like a kind of a ghost, hovering here as an afterthought."

Selfishly, I was happy that he was there. It was our first face-to-face exchange ever, after about a year of long-distance interaction. We had corresponded via E-mail mostly, except for the one day several months before when Morris called to talk. On the phone, we had spoken for a while about his disease and my book. I had thanked him for his many insights, for introducing me to Viktor Frankl and tipping me off to Emerson's dementia. He seemed interested in my aim to write a biography of the disease, and eager to help. We agreed to stay in touch, to keep exchanging ideas.

Now I was eager to continue our discussion. The poster scene, though, was a little too chaotic for a real conversation. We agreed to meet the next day for lunch.

Over sandwiches and coffee at a grill across town, we climbed back into some of our shared curiosities, starting with rehabilitation. He was of course not talking literally about beating this disease with brain exercises, but about minimizing and slowing the cognitive loss by adapting to it.

Why shouldn't Alzheimer's patients get as much conditioning as stroke victims, for example? The disease's ultimate mortality should not automatically annul patients' expectations of living the fullest possible life for the longest possible time.

Alzheimer's is a very slow disease, and there was no particular reason to settle for a passive approach of managing loss—which was often tantamount to hospice care in slow motion. If drugs like Aricept could lead to marginal improvements, it was tantalizing to imagine what a professional rehabilitation program could do. Intensive rehab, in the spirit of what knee and hip surgery patients go through routinely, had just never been considered before in Alzheimer's disease. In the new era of people discovering their disease very early on, the idea made abundant sense.

Morris's proposal was not a first draft. "My previous approach to rehabilitation," he said, "was to substitute intense meaning and emotional organization for [cold analysis], refining your sense of what's important to compensate for your inability to deal with everything.

"I've revised that. If a person has a block in problem solving and it gets too emotional then their memories can get *more* scattered.

"Most of the focus on brain injury has to do with the frontal lobes—auto accidents with younger people and such. People with mild Alzheimer's still have frontal lobes that are functioning very well. They know what they want to do, but they are not able to learn anything from the attempts. There is some work with the Montessori approach to problem solving with people with dementia that's been encouraging. Rather than relearning to pay attention to the problem, I suggest a reeducation vaguely inspired by

Montessori: Do something that's extremely simple, just to get into a confidence mind-set—stringing one or two beads, or something like that. And gradually learn to solve problems in new, simpler ways.

"The spirit of *feng shui* is interesting. I tell other early-stage patients, 'The practical application of my theory is to start getting rid of your clutter,' and this strikes a chord in the way that my other ideas haven't. Eliminate physical clutter as a path to get rid of mental clutter. I'm saying, 'simplify, simplify, simplify'—just like Thoreau."

We talked for two hours. Some of his ideas I understood, some I did not, entirely. Morris sometimes paused for a while, and had to occasionally struggle to stay on track. There was no question that he was slowly succumbing to the disease. Mostly, though, I was left with the impression that he was onto something important, that he *did* understand his own unraveling in a way I would not have ever imagined possible when I first started to learn about this disease. Throughout our lunch, I repeatedly encountered a *frisson* of realization that in several years of research, the most thought-provoking discussions I'd had about Alzheimer's were with one of its victims.

I realized that, in a peculiar way, Morris had rehabilitated *me*—and my understanding of Alzheimer's. When I started my research, I conceived of a book that might, on the one hand, catalogue the horrors of Alzheimer's, and on the other, relay the hopeful story of the race to cure the disease.

I still respected that dichotomy, still feared the disease, and still hoped for a cure, of course—as did Morris. But I also now realized that the story of Alzheimer's is in some ways exactly the opposite of my original premise: It is a condition specific to humans and as old as humanity that, like nothing else, acquaints us with life's richness by ever so gradually drawing down the curtains. Only through modern science has this poignancy been reduced to a plain horror, an utterly unhuman circumstance.

It wouldn't be fair to say that I had transcended the disease in the same way that Morris obviously had, or in the way that Emerson and de Kooning admirably had. After all, I was still only an observer. But it's worth noting that, personally, I migrated over several years' time from morbid fascination and dread of Alzheimer's to a new kind of peace and reconciliation.

As this realization unfolded, I thought of another presentation at the conference, given by the family counselor and author Lisa Snyder. In the Indonesian island of Bali, she reported, there is a powerful myth of life cycles that centers on memory:

Babies are born with no memory. They gather memories as they grow. As they get old they lose these memories so that they can be reborn again in a void.

All of these things I was thinking about as I drove Morris back to his hotel room. I told him again how much I appreciated his ideas, and wished him well.

Then, just before I dropped him off, Morris asked me if we'd ever spoken before today.

EPILOGUE

⌀

I cannot promise you everlasting life, but I can promise you life
right now.

—BRUCE SPRINGSTEEN

Two blocks from my home in Brooklyn is the main entrance to
Prospect Park, an arrow-shaped 526-acre retreat from urban intensity. It is a wondrous place, with a mile-long hilly green meadow, a
great lake, and the last surviving natural forest in Brooklyn. There
is a working nineteenth-century carousel, a band shell for concerts,
picnic tables and barbecue pits, a horse trail, plenty of swing sets,
and wild geese. About six million times a year, people come here
to find themselves.

The park was designed by Calvert Vaux and Frederick Law
Olmsted from 1865 to 1873, just after the pair had completed
their work on Central Park in Manhattan. They had planned to

link the two parks with a ten-mile-long, tree-shadowed "parkway," but could not sell that part of their vision. Still, Olmsted considered his Brooklyn park to be a crowning achievement. "I am prouder of it than anything I have had to do with," he remarked on a later visit.

Olmsted was a champion of urban beautification in the mid-to-late nineteenth century and is now considered the founder of American landscape architecture. He is responsible for an astounding number of treasured urban American refuges, including Chicago's Jackson Park, Boston's Emerald Necklace, and Louisville's Cherokee Park. "The further progress of civilization is to depend mainly upon the influences by which men's minds and characters will be affected while living in large towns," Olmsted argued. A city park, he insisted, must help the resident escape "the devouring eagerness and intellectual strife of town life."

He was abundantly influenced by Emerson, whom he read avidly and met with early in his career. His was an unflinchingly Emersonian notion. "What we want to gain," said Olmsted, "is tranquillity and rest to the mind."

A year or so after Olmsted finished his work on Prospect Park, he moved to Washington, D.C., to design the grounds of the U.S. Capitol, which he worked on for fifteen years, up until 1889. Not long after that, as he neared seventy years old, he started to have memory problems, very subtle at first and then, gradually, more disabling. On the way to pivotal meetings, he would ask his sons to remind him of key names and project details. Then, in North Carolina, he was discovered writing virtually the same letter over and over again to his patron George Vanderbilt, his short-term memory apparently obliterated.

In 1895, at age seventy-three, he wrote his son John, his devoted right hand for twenty years: "I see that I ought no longer to be entrusted to carry on important business for the firm alone." Olmsted retreated into seclusion in Maine (in a house designed by Emerson's cousin, William Ralph Emerson). As John attempted to keep his father tangentially involved in the firm's projects, he made a firm, practical suggestion. "It would be well for you," he wrote his father, "to review the letters we have written you since you went to Deer Isle each time before you write your daily letter to us. . . . [you should] constantly bear in mind that your memory for current events is no longer a working basis for your thoughts."

Things became much darker. Olmsted became paranoid, accusing John of executing a "coup." In 1898, at age seventy-six, it got bad enough that he had to be moved into McLean Asylum, in Waverly, Massachusetts, where he would remain confined until his death in 1903.

Alzheimer's is, in itself, a sort of mental confinement—the sufferer is incarcerated within the collapsing neural structures that he has taken a lifetime to build. But Olmsted, through his own work, inadvertently lived out the metaphor in literal terms. He was imprisoned not just within his own collapsing mind, but also in his own design: Olmsted had created the 275-acre grounds for McLean two decades before. At first, he was bitterly aware of the irony. But by the time he died, he had forgotten not only about his design of McLean, but also about landscapes altogether.

We have not forgotten about him. It has been the great triumph of civilization to compensate for the limits of human life and memory, to extend the fruits of one person's intellect beyond its natural life. Olmsted's magnificent creations have lasted a full century since his decline and are set to last many more. Part of the further progress of civilization will be to help care for those who

ACKNOWLEDGMENTS

◊

There is a woman whom I have never met, whose name I do not know. Let me acknowledge her first, because it was her forgetting that started all this. Eating lunch alone one day in my neighborhood taqueria, I found myself absorbed by a nearby conversation about this woman with early-onset Alzheimer's who could no longer recognize her own husband. I closed my eyes and tried to imagine myself as that husband, and then stumbled back to my office determined to learn more about this disease.

Listening to public radio in my kitchen, I have heard authors from time to time insist that they didn't really choose their book topics—that it's more like the books chose *them*. This is not the sort of thing I expected would ever happen to me.

I am blessed to have Sloan Harris for a literary agent. This book simply could not have happened without him. Much of Sloan's insight into this project, sadly, came out of firsthand experience with the decline of his own grandmother, Louise Walker, to whom I also want to pay tribute.

Bill Thomas, at Doubleday, provided the perfect nest for the fledgling work, and proved to be a masterful and nurturing editor.

I am indebted to Karen Duff, at the Nathan Kline Institute, for her patient tutorials on the molecular biology of Alzheimer's and the politics of that community.

For help unearthing details of Emerson's decline, thanks to Randall Albright, Howard Callaway, Morris Friedell, Roberto Piccoli, and Joel Porte.

Excavation of the ancient history of senility was facilitated by John Baines, Peter Butrica, Lawrence H. Feldman, Joan Ferry, Carol Fleming-Huskisson, François Hinard, Allen Koenigsberg, Julie Langford-Johnson, Russell A. Johnson, James Lawrence, Gert-Jan Lokhorst, David Lupher, Willard L. Marmelzat, Michael Meckler, Ernest Moncada, Tim Parkin, Elaine Perry, George Pesely, James M. Pfundstein, Gil Renberg, Patrick Rourke, Roy Starling, Juergen Stowasser, and Carl Widstrand.

Steven Johnson and James Ryerson, both of *Feed* magazine, spurred the material on memory molecules and Luria's patient S. András Szántó advanced my understanding of the relationship between identity and the artistic process for the chapter on de Kooning.

Thanks to Jed Levine, Tony Yang Lewis, Julie Rosenberg, Stefanie Roth, Judy Joseph, and Irving Brickman for a gentle introduction to the world of caregiving. I am particularly grateful to Irving for his kindness, conferred even as he faced the cancer that ended his life before the completion of this book.

Carla Flaherty generously shared her journal about her father's decline. Dan Paris, Geri Hall, and dozens of other regulars on the Alzheimer List gave me a better education than I could have hoped for. Thanks also to Julie Miller at the Alzheimer Association.

Heiko Braak and Kelly Del Tredici supplied key neuropathological papers, and Dorothy Rice furnished economic data and estimates. For historical guidance, thanks to Matthias M. Weber. Paulette Michaud and Jeffrey Toward were generous to share their transcripts of interviews with early-stage patients. John Trojanowski and Virginia Lee spent some of their valuable time educating a neophyte.

I am grateful to Neil Levi for sharing his translation-in-progress of a biography of Alois Alzheimer. Michael Strong let me read his fascinating dissertation on James Joyce and neuroscience. Richard Gehr opened the door to Nietzsche.

Bruce Feiler, Gersh Kuntzman, Andrew Shapiro, and Eamon Dolan are cherished confidants and advisers. Richard Shenk gave invaluable support. Thanks to Joanne Cohen and Sidney Cohen for reading early drafts. I am also very grateful to Teri Steinberg for her powerful encouragement and insight, and to Kendra Harpster for editorial assistance. Thanks to Apple Computer for so quickly replacing my laptop after it mysteriously caught on fire.

For his music, I thank Keith Jarrett.

For help with the manuscript in its late stages, I am indebted to Andrew Hoffman, Linda Steinman, Roy Kreitner, Daniel Radosh, Gina Duclayan, Tom Inck, Ivan Oransky, and Tom Inglesby. Nick Moore, John Holzman, and Jon Shenk served as much-needed compasses in the harrowing final days.

Word by word, chapter by chapter, my brother Joshua Wolf Shenk helped me make this a much better book.

RESOURCES FOR PATIENTS AND FAMILIES

◦

For families stranded on the island of Alzheimer's disease, the initial feeling can be one of utter desolation. Many soon discover, though, that there are a host of extraordinary provisions available—medical and social services, support groups, books, and products for safety and security—that can make the long stay somewhat less perplexing and more comfortable. Below is a selected guide to some of these aids. (For more information, including medical research updates and links to the surfeit of online resources, visit www.theforgetting.com on the World Wide Web.)

PHONE HOTLINES
Alzheimer's Disease Education and Referral Center, National Institute on Aging
(800) 438-4380
Provides pamphlets and referrals to other agencies.

Alzheimer's Association

(800) 272–3900

Provides information packets and phone numbers for local chapters, which in turn will assist with the complete array of medical and social services.

Safe Return Hotline

(888) 572-8566

Provides information on how to join the Alzheimer's Association's identification-registry program as a precaution for patients who may wander away from home.

American Health Care Association

(202) 842-4444

Provides information on how to choose an assisted living facility or nursing home, and referral to a state chapter that will provide a specific list of local facilities.

BOOKS

Alzheimer's Early Stages: First Steps in Caring and Treatment, by Daniel Kuhn. Publisher's Press, 1999.

There's Still a Person in There: The Complete Guide to Treating and Coping with Alzheimer's, by Michael Castleman, Matthew Naythons, and Dolores Gallagher-Thompson. Putnam, 2000.

The 36-Hour Day: A Family Guide to Caring for Persons with Alzheimer's Disease, Related Dementing Illness, and Memory Loss in Later Life, by Nancy L. Mace and Peter V. Rabins. Johns Hopkins University Press, 1999.

Cooking Well for the Unwell: More Than One Hundred Nutritious Recipes, by Eileen Behan. Hearst Books, 1996.

Elder Law: A Legal and Financial Survival Guide for Caregivers and Seniors, by Peter J. Strauss and Nancy M. Lederman. G. K. Hall & Co., 1996.

The Sunsets of Miss Olivia Wiggins, by Lester L. Laminack. Peachtree Publishers, 1998. (children's book)

Great-Uncle Alfred Forgets, by Ben Schecter. HarperCollins, 1996. (children's book)

Reversing Memory Loss: Proven Methods for Regaining, Strengthening, and Preserving Your Memory, by Vernon H. Mark and Jeffrey P. Mark. Houghton Mifflin, 2000.

Keep Your Brain Alive: 83 Neurobic Exercises, by Lawrence Katz. Workman Publishing, 1999.

PRODUCT CATALOGS
Life Enrichment & Activities
(800) 247-2343
Catalog of products for seniors in decline.

Ageless Design
(561) 745-0210
Products for safety in the home.

SOURCES

◦

By subject, in order of appearance.

Ralph Waldo Emerson

Baker, Carlos. *Emerson Among the Eccentrics: A Group Portrait.* New York: Penguin, 1996.

Bok, Edward. *The Americanization of Edward Bok: An Autobiography.* 1920. Reprint, New York: Pocket Books, 1965.

Cabot, James Elliot. *Memoir of Ralph Waldo Emerson.* 1887. Reprint, New York: AMS Press, 1965.

Emerson, Edward Waldo. *Emerson in Concord: A Memoir.* 1889. Reprint, Detroit: Gale Research Co., 1970.

Emerson, Lydia Jackson. *The Selected Letters of Lydia Jackson Emerson 1802–1892.* Edited by Delores Bird Carpenter. Columbia: University of Missouri Press, 1987.

Emerson, Ralph Waldo. *The Letters of Ralph Waldo Emerson.*

Edited by Eleanor M. Tilton. Vol. 10, *1870–1881.* New York: Columbia University Press, 1995.

———. "Notebook IT." In *The Topical Notebooks of Ralph Waldo Emerson,* edited by Susan Sutton Smith. Columbia: University of Missouri Press, 1990.

———. *Essays: First Series.* 1841. Reprint, Philadelphia: David McKay, 1890.

———. *Natural History of the Intellect.* 1893. Reprint, New York: Solar Press, 1995.

———. *The Journals and Miscellaneous Notebooks of Ralph Waldo Emerson.* Edited by Joel Porte. Cambridge: Harvard University Press, 1982.

———. *The Journals of Ralph Waldo Emerson, 1864–1876.* Edited by Edward Waldo Emerson and Waldo Emerson Forbes. New York: Houghton Mifflin, 1909–1914.

Garnett, Richard. *The Life of Ralph Waldo Emerson.* 1888. Reprint, New York: Haskell House Publishers, 1974.

Gregg, Edith E. W., ed. *The Letters of Ellen Tucker Emerson.* Kent, Ohio: Kent State University Press, 1982.

McAleer, John. *Ralph Waldo Emerson: Days of Encounter.* Boston: Little, Brown, 1984.

Richardson, Robert. *Emerson: The Mind on Fire.* Berkeley: University of California Press, 1995.

Russell, Phillips. *Emerson: The Wisest American.* New York: Brentano's, 1929.

Sealts, Merton M. *Emerson on the Scholar.* Columbia: University of Missouri Press, 1992.

Thayer, James Bradley. *A Western Journey with Mr. Emerson.* 1884. Reprint, Port Washington, N.Y.: Kennikat Press, 1971.

Alois Alzheimer and Emil Kraepelin

Berrios, G. E., and H. L. Freeman. *Alzheimer and the Dementias.* London: Royal Society of Medicine Services Limited, 1991.

Bick, Katherine, *et al. The Early Story of Alzheimer's Disease: Translation of the Historical Papers by Alois Alzheimer, Oskar Fischer, Francesco Bonfiglio, Emil Kraepelin, Gaetano Perusini.* New York: Raven Press, 1987.

Brannon, William L. "Alois Alzheimer (1864–1915) I. Contributions to Neurology and Psychiatry. II. Dementia Before and After Alzheimer: A Brief History." *Journal of the South Carolina Medical Association* 90, no. 9 (September 1994).

Decker, Hannah S. *Freud in Germany.* New York: International Universities Press, 1977.

Lewey, F. H. "Alois Alzheimer." In *The Founders of Neurology.* Springfield, Ill.: Thomas, 1970.

Maurer, Konrad. *A Biography of Alois Alzheimer.* Translated by Neil Levi. New York: Columbia University Press, forthcoming.

——— *et al.* "Auguste D. and Alzheimer's Disease." *Lancet* 349 (24 May 1997).

Weber, Matthias M. "Alois Alzheimer, A Co-worker of Emil Kraepelin." *Journal of Psychiatric Research* 31, no. 6 (1997).

Weindling, Paul. *Health, Race and German Politics Between National Unification and Nazism 1870–1945.* Cambridge: Cambridge University Press, 1989.

Ancient History of Senility

Aristophanes, *The Clouds.* Published as E-text by the Internet Classics Archive, at http://classics.mit.edu/Aristophanes/clouds.html

Berchtold, N. C., and C. W. Cotman. "Evolution in the Conceptualization of Dementia and Alzheimer's Disease: Greco-Roman Period to the 1960s." *Neurobiology of Aging* 19, no. 3 (1998).

Cicero, *Selected Works*. Translated by Michael Grant. New York: Penguin Books, 1960.

Cohen, Gene D. "Historical Views and Evolution of Concepts." In *Alzheimer's Disease,* edited by Barry Reisberg. New York: The Free Press, 1983.

Falkner, Thomas M. and Judith de Luce. *Old Age in Greek and Latin Literature*. Albany: State University of New York Press, 1989.

Finger, Stanley. *Origins of Neuroscience*. New York: Oxford University Press, 1994.

Juvenal. *The Satires of Juvenal*. Translated by C. E. Ramsay. Cambridge, Mass.: Loeb Classical Library/Harvard University Press, 1918.

The New Oxford Annotated Bible. New York: Oxford University Press,

Oxford English Dictionary. Compact Edition. Oxford: Clarendon Press, 1971.

Parkin, Tim. "Out of Sight, Out of Mind: Elderly Members of the Roman Family." In *The Roman Family in Italy,* edited by Beryl Rawson and Paul Weaver. Oxford: Clarendon Press, 1997.

Plato. *Theaetetus*. Published as E-text by Project Gutenberg at www2.cddc.vt.edu/gutenberg/etext99/thtus10.txt

Sahagún, Bernardino de. *General History of the Things of New Spain: Florentine Codex*. Translation. Santa Fe, N.M.: School of American Research and University of Utah, 1950–1982.

The Tale of Sinhue and Other Ancient Egyptian Poems, 1940–1640 B.C. Translated by R. B. Parkinson. Oxford: Oxford University Press, 1997.

Torack, Richard M. "The Early History of Senile Dementia." In *Alzheimer's Disease,* edited by Barry Reisberg. New York: The Free Press, 1983.

Virgil. "Eclogue IX." In *Virgil's Works,* translated by J. W. Mackail. New York: Modern Library, 1950.

Xenophon. *Memorabilia.* Stuttgart: Teubner. 1969.

Ronald Reagan

Altman, Lawrence K. "Reagan's Twilight." *New York Times,* 5 October 1997.

"Maureen Reagan Says She Has Beaten Cancer." Associated Press. 4 May 1998.

Sidey, Hugh. "The Sunset of My Life." *Time,* 14 November 1994.

Strober, Deborah Hart, and Gerald Strober. *Reagan: The Man and His Presidency.* New York: Houghton Mifflin, 1998.

Science of Mind and Memory

Alkon, Daniel L. *Memory's Voice: Deciphering the Mind-Brain Code.* New York: HarperCollins, 1994.

Baddeley, Alan. *Your Memory: A User's Guide.* New York: Macmillan, 1982.

Blakeslee, Dennis. "The Blood-Brain Barrier." Background briefing posted on 5 May 1997 at www.ama-assn.org/special/hiv/newsline/briefing/bbb.htm

Blakeslee, Sandra. "Tests with Rats Offer Clues to Why Memories Change." *Cleveland Plain Dealer,* 25 September 2000.

Bliss, Tim. "The Physiological Basis of Memory." In *From Brains to Consciousness: Essays on the New Sciences of Mind,* edited by Steven Rose. Princeton: Princeton University Press, 1998.

Bolles, Edmund Blair. *Remembering and Forgetting: Inquiries into the Nature of Memory.* New York: Walker and Company, 1988.

Carter, Rita. *Mapping the Mind.* Berkeley: University of California Press, 1998.

Dennett, Daniel C. *Consciousness Explained.* Boston: Little, Brown and Company, 1991.

Goldberg, Stephen. *Clinical Neuroanatomy Made Ridiculously Simple.* Miami: MedMaster, Inc., 1979.

Greenfield, Susan. "How Might the Brain Generate Consciousness." In *From Brains to Consciousness: Essays on the New Sciences of Mind, op. cit.*

Heindel, William C., and Stephen Salloway. "Memory Systems in the Human Brain." *Psychiatric Times,* June 1999.

Johnson, Steven. Interview with Steven Pinker. *Feed* magazine, at www.feedmag.com/re/re181_master.html

Mega, Michael S., *et al.* "The Limbic System: An Anatomic, Phylogenic, and Clinical Perspective." *Journal of Neuropsychiatry* 9 (3): 315–330 (1997).

Meier, Barry. "Industry's Next Growth Sector: Memory Lapses." *New York Times,* 4 April 1999.

Mithen, Steven. *The Prehistory of the Mind: The Cognitive Origins of Art and Science.* London: Thames and Hudson Ltd., 1996.

Noback, Charles R., *et al. The Human Nervous System: Structure and Function.* Philadelphia: Williams and Wilkins, 1996.

Parnavelas, John. "The Human Brain: 100 Billion Connected Cells." In *From Brains to Consciousness: Essays on the New Sciences of Mind, op. cit.*

Pinker, Steven. *How the Mind Works.* New York: W.W. Norton, 1999.

Rhodes, Richard. *Deadly Feasts: The "Prion" Controversy and the Public's Health.* New York: Touchstone, 1998.

Robbins, Trevor. "The Pharmacology of Thought and Emotion." In *From Brains to Consciousness: Essays on the New Sciences of Mind,* op. cit.

Rose, Steven. *The Making of Memory: From Molecules to Mind.* New York: Anchor, 1993.

Rose, Steven P. R. "How Brains Make Memories." In *Memory,* edited by Patricia Fara and Karalyn Patterson. New York: Cambridge University Press, 1998.

Schacter, Daniel L. *Searching for Memory.* New York: Basic Books, 1996.

Scheck, Barry. "Attorney Barry Scheck." *The Connection* (radio program), WBUR, Boston, 16 March 2000.

Sejnowski, Terrence J. "Memory and Neural Networks." In *Memory,* op. cit.

Selkoe, Dennis J. "Alzheimer's Disease: A Central Role for Amyloid." *Journal of Neuropathology and Experimental Neurology* 53, no. 5 (September 1994).

Smith, A. David. "Ageing of the Brain: Is Mental Decline Inevitable?" In *From Brains to Consciousness: Essays on the New Sciences of Mind,* op. cit.

Squire, Larry R. "Memory and Brain Systems." In *From Brains to Consciousness: Essays on the New Sciences of Mind,* op. cit.

Strong, Michael. "When Language Goes on Holiday: *Finnegans Wake,* Neuroscience, and Models of Subjectivity." Dissertation, University of Pennsylvania, forthcoming.

Tanner, J. M. *Fetus into Man: Physical Growth from Conception to Maturity.* Cambridge, Mass.: Harvard University Press, 1990.

Wilson, Barbara A. "When Memory Fails." In *Memory,* op. cit.

S., The Man with the Perfect Memory

Luria, A. R. *The Mind of a Mnemonist: A Little Book About a Vast Memory.* Translated from the Russian by Lynn Solotaroff. Cambridge: Harvard University Press, 1968.

The History of Disease

Aronowitz, Robert A. *Making Sense of Illness: Science, Society, and Disease.* New York: Cambridge University Press, 1998.

Gross, Charles G. *Brain Vision Memory: Tales in the History of Neuroscience.* Cambridge, Mass.: MIT Press, 1998.

Porter, Roy. *The Greatest Benefit to Mankind: A Medical History of Humanity.* New York: W.W. Norton, 1997.

Quétel, Claude. *The History of Syphilis.* Translated by Judith Braddock and Brian Pike. Baltimore: Johns Hopkins University Press, 1992.

Rosenberg, Charles E., and Janet Golden, eds. *Framing Disease: Studies in Cultural History.* New Brunswick, N.J.: Rutgers University Press, 1992.

Shorter, Edward. *A History of Psychiatry: From the Era of the Asylum to the Age of Prozac.* New York: John Wiley & Sons, 1997.

Temkin, Oswei. *The Double Face of Janus and Other Essays in the History of Medicine.* Baltimore: Johns Hopkins University Press, 1977.

Shift from "Senility" to "Alzheimer's Disease"

Cecil, Russell L., and Robert F. Loeb. *A Textbook of Medicine.* Philadelphia: W.B. Saunders, 1955.

Dillman, Rob. *Alzheimer's Disease: The Concept of Disease and the Construction of Medical Knowledge.* Amsterdam: Thesis Publishers, 1990.

Fox, Patrick. "From Senility to Alzheimer's Disease: The Rise of the Alzheimer's Disease Movement." *Milbank Quarterly* 67, Issue 1 (1989).

HISTNEUR-L, The History of Neuroscience Internet Forum: http:www.melsch.ucla.edu/sam/bri/archives/histneur.htm

Neumann, Meta A., and Robert Cohn. "Incidence of Alzheimer's Disease in a Large Mental Hospital." *Archives of Neurology and Psychiatry* 69 (May 1953).

White, Lon. "Alzheimer's Disease: The Evolution of a Diagnosis." *Public Health Reports,* November-December 1997.

Alzheimer's Caregiving

Henderson, Cary Smith. *Partial View: An Alzheimer's Journal.* Dallas: Southern Methodist University Press, 1998.

Kuhn, Daniel. *Alzheimer's Early Stages: First Steps in Caring and Treatment.* Salt Lake City: Publishers Press, 1999.

Mace, Nancy L., and Peter V. Rabins. *The 36-Hour Day.* New York: Warner, 1992.

Michaud, Paulette. *Early Stages: Changing Our Views of Alzheimer's.* New York: Alzheimer's Association, 1998.

Murphy, Beverly Bigtree. *He Used to Be Somebody.* Boulder, Colo.: Gibbs Associates, 1995.

Snyder, Lisa. *Speaking Our Minds: Personal Reflections from Individuals with Alzheimer's.* New York: W.H. Freeman, 1999.

Stephenson, Crocker. "The Vanishing Man." *Milwaukee Journal Sentinel,* 27 December 1998.

King Lear

Bullough, Geoffrey, ed. *Narrative and Dramatic Sources of Shakespeare.* Vol. 8. New York: Columbia University Press, 1973.

Bullough, Geoffrey. *"King Lear* and the Annesley Case: A Reconsideration." *Festchrift Rudolf Stamm.* Munich: Francke Verlag Bern, 1969.

Shakespeare, William. *King Lear.* Edited by Alfred Harbage. New York: Penguin Books, 1970.

———. *King Lear.* Edited by Kenneth Muir. London: Methuen & Co., 1978.

Morris Friedell

The essays "Introduction to Myself and My Plight," "Incipient Dementia: A Victim's Perspective," "Love in the Twilight Zone," and "The Road to Alzheimer's" are published, among many others, on Morris's Internet home page: http://members.aol.com/MorrisFF.

Human Suffering

Becker, Ernest. *The Denial of Death.* New York: Free Press, 1973.

Frankl, Viktor E. *Man's Search for Meaning.* New York: Washington Square Press, 1985.

Post, Stephen G. *The Moral Challenge of Alzheimer's Disease.* Baltimore: Johns Hopkins University Press, 1995.

Sontag, Susan. *Illness as Metaphor & AIDS and Its Metaphors.* New York: Anchor Books, 1990.

Alzheimer's Disease and Science

Baddeley, Alan D., Barbara A. Wilson, and Fraser N. Watts, eds. *Handbook of Memory Disorders.* New York: John Wiley & Sons, 1998.

Braak, Heiko, and Eva Braak. "Temporal Sequence of Alzheimer's Disease-Related Pathology." Vol. 14. *Cerebral Cortex.* Edited by Peters and Morrison. New York: Kluwer Academic/Plenum Publishers, 1999.

Clark, Cheryl. "Irony and Illness Hit Alzheimer's Researcher." *San Diego Union-Tribune,* 6 April 1995.

Dalton, Rex. "Researchers Caught in Dispute Over Transgenic Mice Patents." *Nature,* 23 March 2000.

Duff, Karen. "Alzheimer Transgenic Mouse Models Come of Age." *Trends in Neurosciences* 20, no. 7 (July 20, 1997).

———. "Curing Amyloidosis: Will It Work in Humans?" *Trends in Neurosciences* 22, no. 11 (November 1999).

Folstein, M. F., *et al.* "Mini-Mental State: A Practical Method for Grading the State of Patients for the Clinician." *Journal of Psychiatric Research* 12, pp. 196–198 (1975).

Franssen, Emile H., and Barry Reisberg. "Neurologic Markers of the Progression of Alzheimer's Disease." *International Psychogeriatrics* 9, suppl. 1 (1997).

Franssen, Emile H., *et al.* "Utility of Developmental Reflexes in the Differential Diagnosis and Prognosis of Incontinence in Alzheimer's Disease." *Journal of Geriatric Psychiatry and Neurology* 10 (January 1997).

Hyman, B. T. "The Neuropathological Diagnosis of Alzheimer's Disease: Clinical-Pathological Studies." *Neurobiology of Aging* 18, no. S4 (1997).

Iqbal, Khalid, *et al. Alzheimer's Disease and Related Disorders: Etiology, Pathogenesis and Therapeutics.* New York: John Wiley & Sons, 1999.

Itzhaki, Ruth F. "Viruses and Alzheimer's Disease." *Science Spectra* no. 14 (1998).

Katzman, Robert, and Katherine Bick. *Alzheimer's Disease: The Changing View.* New York: Academic Press, 2000.

Khachaturian, Zaven S. "Plundered Memories." *The Sciences,* July/August 1997.

Langreth, Robert. "To Fight Alzheimer's, Drug Firms Place Bets on an Unproven Theory." *Wall Street Journal,* 8 July 1999.

Marshall, Eliot. "Allen Roses: From 'Street Fighter' to Corporate Insider." *Science,* 15 May 1998.

Marx, Jean. "New 'Alzheimer's Mouse' Produced." *Science,* 11 October 1996.

Masters, Colin L., and Konrad Beyreuther. "Science, Medicine, and the Future: Alzheimer's Disease." *British Medical Journal,* 7 February 1998.

National Institute on Aging. *Alzheimer's Disease: Unraveling the Mystery.* October 1995. Available at www.alzheimers.org/unravel.html

Nelson, Peter. Interview with Karen Duff, 24 May 1999. Available at www.alzforum.org/members/forums/interview/karen_duff. html

Pollen, Daniel A. *Hannah's Heirs: The Quest for the Genetic Origins of Alzheimer's Disease.* New York: Oxford University Press, 1996.

Reisberg, Barry. *Alzheimer's Disease: The Standard Reference.* New York: Free Press, 1983.

———, *et al.* "Towards a Science of Alzheimer's Disease Management: A Model Based Upon Current Knowledge of Retrogenesis." *International Psychogeriatrics* 11, no. 1 (1999).

———. "Retrogenesis: Clinical, Physiologic, and Pathologic Mechanisms in Brain Aging, Alzheimer's and Other Dementing Processes." *European Archive of Psychiatry in Clinical Neurosciences* 249, suppl. 3 (1999).

Rovner, Sandy. "Aluminum Foiled." *Washington Post,* 9 March 1984.

Singer, Dorothy G., and Tracey A. Revenson. *How a Child Thinks: A Piaget Primer.* New York: Plume, 1978.

Longevity

Alexander, Brian. "Don't Die, Stay Pretty." *Wired,* January 2000.

Anderson, Robert N. "United States Abridged Life Tables, 1996." National Vital Statistics Reports, 24 December 1998.

Brookmeyer, Ron, *et al.* "Projections of Alzheimer's Disease in the United States and the Public Health Impact of Delaying Disease Onset." *American Journal of Public Health,* September 1998.

Eckholm, Erik. "An Aging Nation Grapples with Care for Old and Ill." *New York Times,* 27 March 1990. *(Note:* This is the first of four articles in the series: "Care of the Elderly; Private Burdens, Public Choices.")

Kirkland, Richard I. "Why We Will Live Longer . . . and What It Will Mean." *Fortune,* 21 February 1994.

Kristof, Nicholas D. "Aging World, New Wrinkles." *New York Times,* 22 September 1996.

Moody, Harry R. "Four Scenarios for an Aging Society." *The Hastings Center Report* 24, no. 5 (September 1994).

Olshansky, S. Jay, Bruce A. Carnes, and Christine K. Cassel. "The Aging of the Human Species." *Scientific American,* April 1993.

Olshansky, S. Jay, Bruce A. Carnes, and Douglas Grahn. "Confronting the Boundaries of Human Longevity." *American Scientist,* 11 January 1998.

Population Institute. "1998 World Population Overview and Outlook 1999." December 30, 1998. Available at http://www.populationinstitute.org/overview98.html

Rice, Dorothy P., *et al.* "The Economic Burden of Alzheimer's Disease Care." *Health Affairs,* Summer 1993.

U.S. Census Bureau. *Sixty-Five Plus in the United States.* May 1995.

———. "Estimated Number of People with Alzheimer's Now and Projections for 2025 (Broken Down by State)." Available at www.census.gov/population/www/projections/pp147.html

West, Maureen. "Turning Back Time." *Denver Rocky Mountain News,* 20 July 1999.

Jonathan Swift

Ehrenpreis, Irvin. *The Personality of Jonathan Swift.* Cambridge: Harvard University Press, 1958.

Glendinning, Victoria. *Jonathan Swift.* New York: Henry Holt, 1998.

Swift, Jonathan. *Gulliver's Travels.* 1726. Reprint, Boston: Houghton Mifflin, 1960.

———. *Prose Writings of Swift.* Chosen and Arranged by Walter Lewin. London: Walter Scott, Ltd., 1896.

Wilde, W. R. *The Closing Years of Dean Swift's Life.* Dublin: Hodges and Smith, 1849.

Willem de Kooning

Abbe, Mary. "Portrait of the Artist as an Old Man." *(Minneapolis) Star Tribune,* 4 February 1996.

de Kooning, Willem. *The Late Paintings: The 1980s.* San Francisco: San Francisco Museum of Modern Art/Minneapolis: Walker Art Center, 1995.

Espinel, Carlos Hugo. "De Kooning's Late Colours and Forms: Dementia, Creativity, and the Healing Power of Art." *Lancet,* 20 April 1996.

Larson, Kay. "Alzheimer's Expressionism." *Village Voice,* 31 May 1994.

Pepper, Curtis Bill. "The Indomitable De Kooning." *New York Times,* 20 November 1983.

Scaruffi, Piero. "Thinking About Thought." *Science's Last Frontiers: Consciousness, Life and Meaning.* Available at www.thymos.com/tat/consc2.html

Mnemonics

Yates, Frances A. *The Art of Memory.* Chicago: University of Chicago Press, 1966.

Frederick Law Olmsted

Roper, Laura Wood. *FLO: A Biography of Frederick Law Olmsted.* Baltimore: Johns Hopkins University Press, 1983.

Rybczynski, Witold. *A Clearing in the Distance: Frederick Law Olmsted and America in the Nineteenth Century.* New York: Scribner, 1999.

Stevenson, Elizabeth. *Park Maker: A Life of Frederick Law Olmsted.* New York: Macmillan, 1977.

Soliloquies

Page 9: Michaud, Paulette. *Early Stages: Changing Our Views of Alzheimer's.* New York: Alzheimer's Association, 1998.

Page 27: Michaud, Paulette. *Early Stages: Changing Our Views of Alzheimer's.* New York: Alzheimer's Association, 1998.

Page 43: Henderson, Cary Smith. *Partial View: An Alzheimer's Journal.* Dallas: Southern Methodist University Press, 1998.

Page 61: Snyder, Lisa. *Speaking Our Minds: Personal Reflections from Individuals with Alzheimer's.* New York: W.H. Freeman, 1999.

Page 71: Rose, Larry. *Show Me the Way to Go Home.* Forest Knolls, California: Elder Books, 1995.

Page 85: Toward, Jeffrey. Interviews with early-stage patients (unpublished). Houston: University of Texas Center on Aging, 1997.

Page 111: Snyder, Lisa. *Speaking Our Minds: Personal Reflections from Individuals with Alzheimer's.* New York: W.H. Freeman, 1999.

Page 131: Originally posted on Alzheimer List, 1998, at http://www.adrc.wustl.edu/alzheimer

Page 147: Originally posted on Alzheimer List, 1998.

Page 161: Originally posted on Alzheimer List, 1998.

Page 177: Originally posted on Alzheimer List, 1999.

Page 191: Originally posted on Alzheimer List, 1999.

Page 215: Originally posted on Alzheimer List, 1998.

Page 227: Petrovski, Sue. *Return Journey.* Book in progress.

Page 241: Morris Friedell, "The Loneliness of a Person with Early Alzheimer's Disease," published online at http://members.aol.com/MorrisFF/

INDEX